No Stones Left Unturned

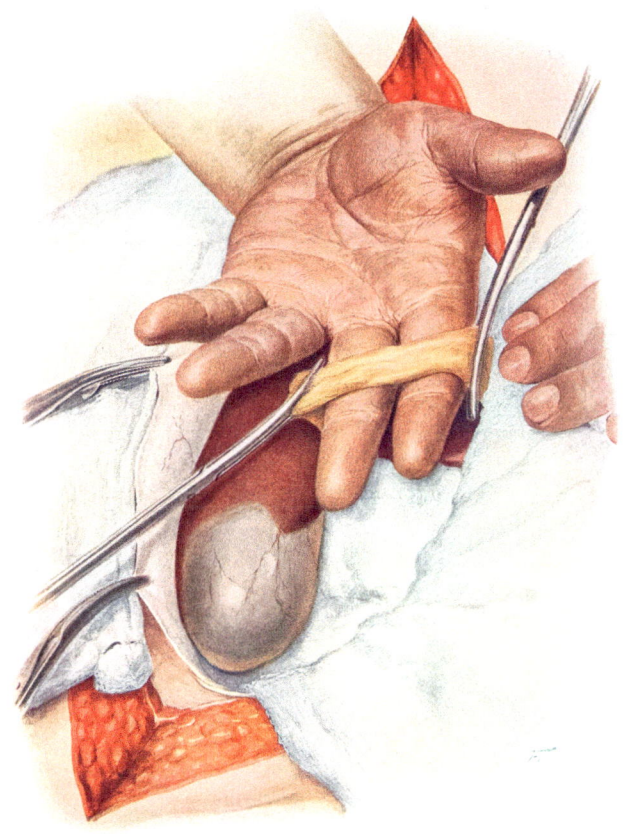

George Berci · Frederick L. Greene

No Stones Left Unturned

Hans Kehr and His Contributions to Biliary
Surgery from Inception to Worldwide
Application in the Modern Era
of Laparoscopic Surgery

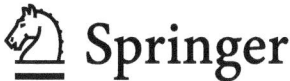

George Berci
Department of Surgery
Cedars-Sinai Medical Center
Los Angeles, CA
USA

Frederick L. Greene
Levine Cancer Institute
Charlotte, NC
USA

ISBN 978-3-030-76844-7   ISBN 978-3-030-76845-4   (eBook)
https://doi.org/10.1007/978-3-030-76845-4

© The Editor(s) (if applicable) and The Author(s), under exclusive license to Springer Nature Switzerland AG 2021, corrected publication 2021
This work is subject to copyright. All rights are solely and exclusively licensed by the Publisher, whether the whole or part of the material is concerned, specifically the rights of translation, reprinting, reuse of illustrations, recitation, broadcasting, reproduction on microfilms or in any other physical way, and transmission or information storage and retrieval, electronic adaptation, computer software, or by similar or dissimilar methodology now known or hereafter developed.
The use of general descriptive names, registered names, trademarks, service marks, etc. in this publication does not imply, even in the absence of a specific statement, that such names are exempt from the relevant protective laws and regulations and therefore free for general use.
The publisher, the authors and the editors are safe to assume that the advice and information in this book are believed to be true and accurate at the date of publication. Neither the publisher nor the authors or the editors give a warranty, expressed or implied, with respect to the material contained herein or for any errors or omissions that may have been made. The publisher remains neutral with regard to jurisdictional claims in published maps and institutional affiliations.

This Springer imprint is published by the registered company Springer Nature Switzerland AG
The registered company address is: Gewerbestrasse 11, 6330 Cham, Switzerland

This book is dedicated to the memory of
Leon Morgenstern, MD, FACS
(1919–2012)
Professor of Surgery, University of California, Los Angeles
Chairman, Department of Surgery
Cedars Sinai Medical Center
Surgeon, Scholar, Educator, and Mentor
A Friend to both of us, who recognized the contributions of Hans Kehr.

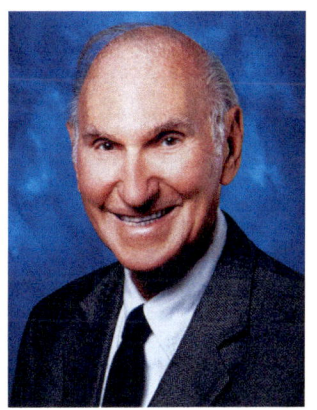

Preface

Knowledge is learning something new every day;
Wisdom is letting go of something every day. –Zen Proverb

From antiquity until now, the beginning of the third decade of the twenty-first century, the application of surgical principles for treatment of biliary stone disease has depended on newer technologies that have allowed a safer and more precise approach to the biliary system. The introduction of open surgical techniques is the bedrock of this surgical journey and is highlighted in this book through the unique contributions of Hans Kehr working in the German School of Surgery. From the late nineteenth century until the latter part of the twentieth century, the principles of open surgery were supported by tremendous improvements in anesthetic care and the application of imaging techniques not dreamed of by Kehr and his colleagues.

In the late 1980s, the laparoscope ushered in a virtual revolution in the approach to gallbladder pathology and biliary stone disease. This "disruptive" technology created an upheaval in every facet of surgery—working through scopes, visualization from operating room monitors, and application of surgical strategies that contributed to patient improvements but, unfortunately, in many cases to detrimental outcomes. Training in these newer, non-traditional approaches also suffered in that adherence to principles of open surgery was frequently eschewed. The application of operative biliary imaging, although advocated by some, was not adhered to by many others.

This incredible story, launched by Hans Kehr and Carl Langenbuch in Germany, continues to unfold in operating suites around the world today. This book is a tribute to early pioneers and later innovators in applications of surgical principles for biliary stone disease. It is also written as a challenge to all surgeons applying these principles to approach the biliary system with the safest and most appropriate technical support. This book is also written as a challenge to all those involved in the training of future generations of surgeons in the hope that critical standards in biliary surgical management will be promulgated and highlighted.

To enhance this book, we have invited current surgical leaders who played a vital part in the modern management of biliary stone disease to contribute their perceptions, wisdom, and recommendations for the future to this book. It is our hope that by highlighting the contributions of both early surgical giants and modern surgical leaders, a coherent message will evolve that current surgical management, while good, is not perfect. We hope that you, our readers, will benefit from this historical approach that is carried forward to current-day management. We hope we will all benefit from the lessons learned. Finally, we hope that this treatise stimulates all to discover ways to make the surgical management of biliary stone disease even better.

Los Angeles, CA, USA George Berci
Charlotte, NC, USA Frederick L. Greene

January 2021

Acknowledgement

The authors are indebted to the skill, tenacity, and dedication of Susan Frederick and Marc Arizmendez, without whose support this book would not have been completed. Susan worked through many manuscript drafts to coordinate and assemble our work between Los Angeles and Charlotte during this time of pandemic. Marc, with his strong skill set in photography and technology, coordinated our manuscript production as well as our many ZOOM deliberations and was instrumental in bringing the illustrations, especially those from the original Kehr edition, to a new generation of readers. Both Susan and Marc worked long hours and through many weekends in the creation of *No Stones Left Unturned*. To them, we are forever grateful.

Introduction

January 2021

The story of cholecystectomy presents a rich tableau of adventuresome surgeons and brilliant innovators. In the late nineteenth century, giants such Hans Kehr advanced the field through impeccable anatomic studies which he and his collaborators selflessly shared with an international audience. A century later, it was fitting that the minimally invasive removal of the gallbladder was the single most impactful advance of that surgical revolution.

This volume, thoughtfully curated by two eminent surgical scholars, provides perhaps the most complete history of the field. In the telling, Drs. Berci and Greene have enlisted a remarkable panel of distinguished colleagues from around the world. Virtually, every important element of surgical practice is discussed with wisdom and perspective: the resourcefulness of developing novel optics and instruments on "the fly"; the integration of new imaging capabilities into pre-operative assessments and intraoperative management; the challenge of educating prideful senior surgeons, ill at ease with the distance imposed by a laparoscope; the introduction of progressively more elegant ex vivo modules to train inexperienced juniors with limited open operative experience; and, finally, the never-ending task of ensuring the safety of one of the most common operations performed in the world, yet one with a persistent, if small, risk of life-altering injury to the biliary ducts.

And one more thing, it is a joy to read. The accounts the contributors share are deeply personal and inspiring. They recapture in detail the excitement they experienced as the field was catapulted forward, offering millions of patients new options for health and longevity. It is a story worth telling – and remembering.

Bruce L. Gewertz, MD, FACS
Professor of Surgery Chair
Department of Surgery Cedars Sinai Medical Center
Los Angeles, California, USA

Contents

Part I Kehr and His Textbook

1. **The History of Biliary Stone Disease** ... 3
   References ... 5

2. **Professor Dr. Hans Kehr (1862–1916)** ... 7
   References ... 10

3. **Translation of Professor Dr. Hans Kehr** ... 11
   Instruments ... 18
   Description of Surgical Cases (Bilingual) Translation ... 20

4. **The Anatomy and Variations of Important Structures** ... 27

5. **Biliary Stones** ... 33
   Summarized Case Report ... 37
   Gallbladders with Carcinomas ... 46
   Preoperative Position ... 48

6. **Surgery** ... 49
   Summarized Detail of 68 Operated Cases ... 53
   Mortality: 7 Cases (9.3%) ... 53

Part II The Gallbladder and Adjacent Structures

7. **History of Endoscopy** ... 57
   Maximilian Nitze (1849–1906), Germany ... 59
   Hans Christian Jacobeus [2] (1879–1937), Sweden ... 60
   References ... 60

8. **Early Biliary Surgeons** ... 61
   References ... 63

9. **Early American Surgeons** ... 65
   References ... 68

10. **Endoscopy** ... 69
    References ... 71

11. **Laparoscopy** ... 73
    Heinz Kalk (1895–1973), Germany ... 74
    John Ruddock (1891–1964), USA ... 74
    References ... 74

12	**Advances in Visualization for Laparoscopic Surgery**	75
	References	78

13	**Laparoscopic Cholecystectomies**	79
	References	83

14	**Cholangiography in the Operating Room**	85

J. Andrew Hamlin

Standard Operative Cholangiography [6]	86
Operative Fluoro-Cholangiography	87
Benefits of the Cholangiogram	88
Biliary Ductal Anatomy	88
Biliary Duct Stones	89
References	90

15	**Bile Duct Injuries**	93
	References	96

16	**Common Bile Duct Stones and Choledocholithotomy**	97
	CBD Stones	97
	References	100

17	**Laparoscopic Cholecystectomy: Introduction, Uptake, Maturity, and Impact on Surgical Practice—Personal Reflections from the Shop Floor**	101

Alfred Cuschieri

Introduction	101
Nomenclature and Origin of Laparoscopic Surgery/Cholecystectomy	102
General Considerations	103
Initial Nosocomial Surgical Epidemic	105
Techniques of Laparoscopic Cholecystectomy	108
Patients with Symptomatic Gallstones and Ductal Calculi	109
Day Case/Ambulatory LC	110
Bleeding Complications Associated with LC	111
Training and Simulation	112
Impact of LC on Surgical Practice across the Specialties	112
Advent of Robotically Assisted Laparoscopic Surgery	114
What Next?	114
References	115

Part III Commentaries

18	**Commentaries**	121
	Commentary	121

Desmond H. Birkett

Teaching the Laparoscopic Common Bile Duct Exploration to
Acute Care Surgeons ... 123

Matthew Bloom

Commentary: Berci-Greene "No Stones Left Unturned" Kehr Book ... 125

L. Michael Brunt

The Trajectory of Biliary Surgery: Personal Reflections ... 127

Daniel J. Deziel

Commentary ... 131

Robert Fitzgibbons and Charles Filipi

Laparoscopic Cholecystectomy: At the Beginning…1989–1990 ... 133

John G. Hunter

Personal Perspective/Experience—In This Surgical Space 135
Joseph B. Petelin
Each Major Advance in Biliary Surgery Needed a
New Way of Teaching 139
Edward H. Phillips
Biliary Surgery: A Story of Innovation and Change 143
Jeffrey L. Ponsky
Commentary 145
Walter J. Pories
For Me, It Started with Diagnostic Laparoscopy 147
Barry Salky
Commentary 149
Jozsef Sandor
Commentary 153
Nathaniel J. Soper
A Personal Glimpse at Bile Duct Injury During
Laparoscopic Cholecystectomy 157
Steven M. Strasberg
My "Rebirth" as a "Laparoscopic" Surgeon: And What that
Means for Surgeons Today 159
Lee Swanström
Technology Advance in Surgery in Both Worlds: Long-Term
Personal Overview 161
Tehemton Erach Udwadia
Reflections of a Trainee During the Laparoscopic
Cholecystectomy Revolution 1989–1992 165
Sherry M. Wren
References 167

Part IV Looking to the Future

19 Epilogue 171
Recommendations for the Future of Surgical Treatment of
Biliary Stone Disease 171
Training Courses 171
Intraoperative Cholangiography, Anatomy, Bile Leakage,
and Stone Identification 172
Conclusion 174
References 174

Correction to: No Stones Left Unturned C1

Index 175

Contributors

Desmond H. Birkett, MD, FACS, FRCS Lahey Hospital and Medical Center, Burlington, MA, USA

Tufts University School of Medicine, Boston, MA, USA

Matthew Bloom, MD, FACS Cedars Sinai Medical Center, Los Angeles, CA, USA

L. Michael Brunt, MD, FACS Section of Minimally Invasive Surgery, Washington University Institute for Minimally Invasive Surgery, Washington University School of Medicine, St. Louis, MO, USA

Daniel J. Deziel, MD, FACS Department of Surgery, Rush University Medical Center, Chicago, IL, USA

Charles Filipi, MD, FACS Department of Surgery, Creighton University Medical School, Omaha, NB, USA

Robert Fitzgibbons Jr, MD, FACS Department of Surgery, Creighton University Medical School, Omaha, NB, USA

John G. Hunter, MD, FACS, FRCS Edin (hon) Oregon Health Science University Health, Portland, OR, USA

Joseph B. Petelin, MD, FACS University of Kansas School of Medicine, Shawnee Mission, KS, USA

Edward H. Phillips, MD, FACS Division of General Surgery, Department of Surgery, Cedars Sinai Medical Center, Los Angeles, CA, USA

Jeffrey L. Ponsky, MD, FACS Cleveland Clinic Lerner College of Medicine, Case Western Reserve University, Cleveland, OH, USA

Walter J. Pories, MD, FACS, Colonel MC USA (RET.) Biochemistry and Kinesiology, Metabolic Surgery Research Group, Brody School of Medicine, East Carolina University, Greenville, NC, USA

Barry Salky, MD, FACS Department of Surgery, Mount Sinai Health System, New York, NY, USA

Jozsef Sandor, MD, PhD, FACS (Hon) Semmelweis University, Budapest, Hungary

Nathaniel J. Soper, MD, FACS Department of Surgery, University of Arizona College of Medicine-Phoenix, Phoenix, AZ, USA

Steven M. Strasberg, MD, FACS Section of HPB Surgery, Washington University, St Louis, MO, USA

Lee Swanström, MD, FACS Oregon Health Sciences University, Portland, OR, USA

Tehemton Erach Udwadia, MS, FCPS Grant Medical College and J.J. Hospital, Mumbai, India

Breach Candy Hospital and Research Center, Mumbai, India

Department of MAS, Hinduja Hospital and Research Center, Mumbai, India

Center of Excellence for Minimal Access Surgery, Mumbai, India

Sherry M. Wren, MD, FACS Center for Innovation and Global Health, Stanford University, Palo Alto Veterans Hospital, Stanford, CA, USA

Special Contributing Authors

Sir Alfred Cuschieri, MD, FRCS, FACS (Hon) Professor of Surgery Molecular Oncology and Surgical Technology, University of Dundee, Dundee, UK

Italian Government Ministry of Universities and Research (MUIR) in Surgery and Nanotechnology, Sant'Anna Advanced School for University Studies and Research, Pisa, Italy

University of St Andrews, St Andrews, UK

PI Medical Robotics and Technology Group, Institute for Medical Science & Technology (IMSaT), University of Dundee, Dundee, UK

J. Andrew Hamlin, MD, FACR Emeritus, Department of Radiology, Cedars Sinai Medical Center, Los Angeles, CA, USA

Part I
Kehr and His Textbook

The History of Biliary Stone Disease

Abstract

While the recognition of gallstones as an abnormality within the human body dates back at least to the fifth century, the treatment of symptomatic gallstone disease remained primitive and ineffective until the eighteenth century. Thudichum proposed a two-stage elective cholecystostomy. Dr. John Stough Bobbs performed the first cholecystotomy. J. Marion Sims must be credited with designing, perfecting, and performing the first cholecystostomy. Later in the nineteenth century Kehr and Langenbuch would usher in the era of open cholecystectomy.

Keywords

Biliary history · Cholecystostomy
Cholecystotomy · Surgical history

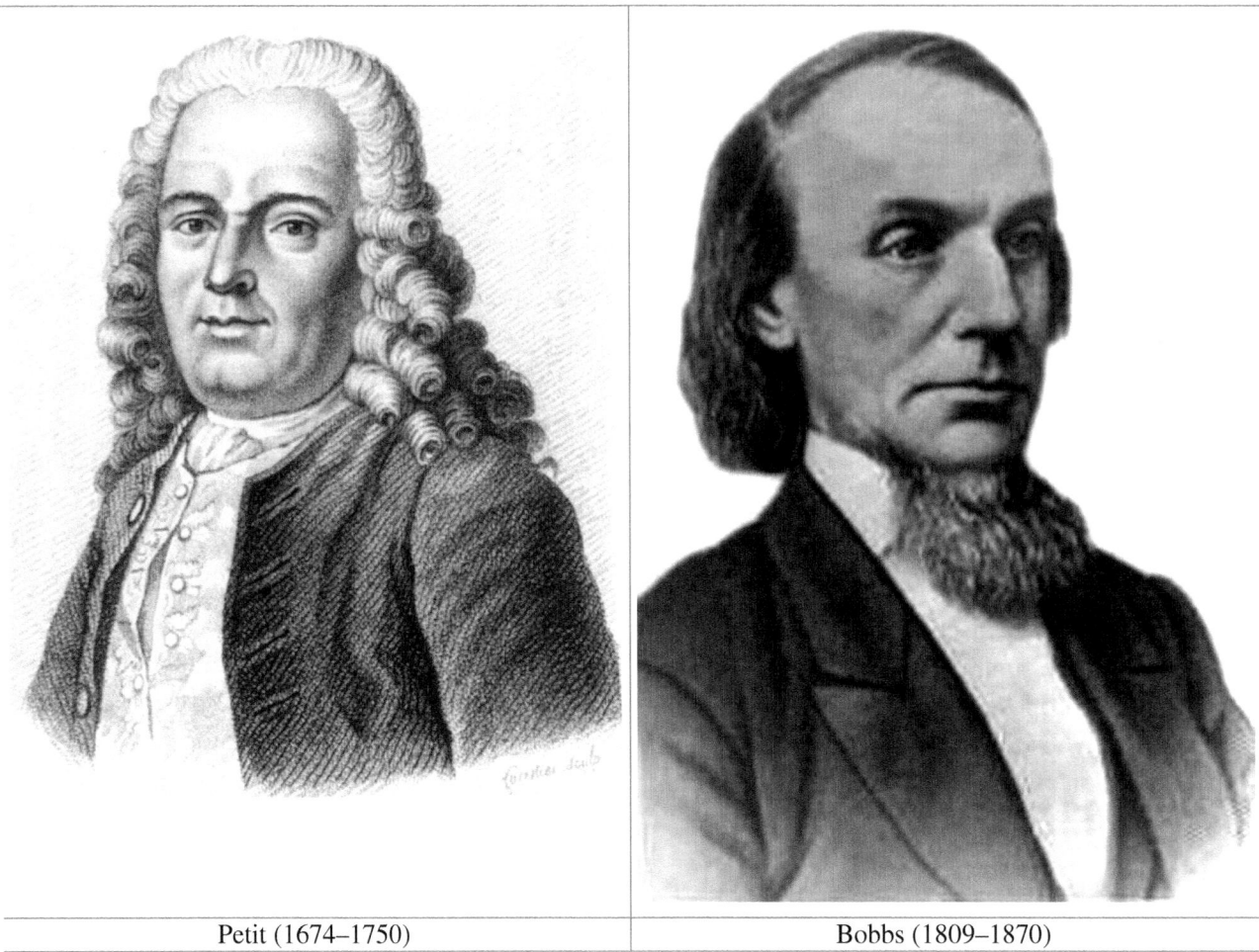

| Petit (1674–1750) | Bobbs (1809–1870) |

The first account of gallstones, given in 1420 by a Florentine pathologist, Antonio Benevieni [1] reported a woman who died with abdominal pain. Centuries followed with ever-increasing recognition of biliary colic. The description of these clinical scenarios flooded the medical literature with numerous physicians and surgeons, including Francis Glisson in 1658 [2], reporting similar cases of biliary colic [3].

The recognition of gallstones as an abnormality within the human body dates back at least to the fifth century. Andreas Vesalius (1514–1564) [4, 5] established that gallstones were associated with disease and could cause jaundice. Morgagni [6], late in the eighteenth century [5], established a correlation between the clinical course and the autopsy findings in a group of patients with obstructive jaundice.

In 1676, a physician by the name of Joenisius [6] removed gallstones from a spontaneous biliary fistula of the abdominal wall that formed after rupture of an abscess and, thereby, has been credited with the first successful cholecystolithotomy. During this time, two animal experiments by Zambecarri in 1630 [7] and Teckoff in 1667 [8] had shown that the gallbladder was not essential to life. Moreover, physicians were of the opinion that the gallbladder itself gave rise to stones. The first interaction of gallstones and surgery dates back to 1687 when Stal Pert Von der Wiel, while performing surgery on a patient with purulent peritonitis, accidentally found gallstones [9]. Nonetheless, the treatment of symptomatic gallstone disease remained primitive and ineffective until the eighteenth century.

Jean-Louis Petit (1674–1750), the founder of gallbladder surgery, suggested the removal of gallstones and drainage of the gallbladder, thus creating a fistula in patients with empyema, which he successfully performed in 1743 [10]. Petit's rigid criteria of surgical intervention were modified over the years. It included skin stimulants to provoke adhesion of the gallbladder to the abdominal wall and subsequent introduction of an indwelling trocar to remove stones and bile from the adhered gallbladder to minimize peritonitis. Thus, this procedure was the prevailing operative management until 1859, when J. L.W. Thudichum proposed a two-stage elective cholecystotomy [11]. In the first stage, the inflamed gallbladder was sewed to the anterior abdominal wall through a small incision, which served as a route for the removal of gallstones at a later date.

Several years later, on July 15, 1867, Dr John Stough Bobbs (1809–1870) from Indianapolis, Indiana, found an inflamed and adhered sac containing "several solid ordinary rifle bullet-like structures" while operating on a patient with a suspected ovarian cyst [12]. He opened the sac, which incidentally happened to be the gallbladder packed with multiple gallstones. He removed the gallstones and left the gallbladder in the abdomen after closing the defect in the gallbladder (cholecystotomy). The patient recovered and outlived Dr. Bobbs.

J. Marion Sims (1831–1883) [13] must be credited with designing, perfecting, and performing the first cholecystostomy on a 45-year-old woman with obstructive jaundice in 1878. Though the patient died on the eighth postoperative day due to massive internal hemorrhage, it paved the way for Theodor Kocher to perform the first successful cholecystostomy in June 1878 [14].

References

1. Ammon H V., Hofmann AF. The Langenbuch Paper. I. An Historical Perspective and Comments of the Translators. Gastroenterology. 1983;85(6):1426–1430. https://doi.org/10.1016/S0016-5085(83)80028-6.
2. Grey Turner G. The history of gall-bladder surgery. Brit Med J. 1939;1(4078):464–465.
3. Praderi RC, Hess, W.A. Brief History of Biliopancreatic Diseases and Their Treatment, Part XII, in: Hess and Berci, *Textbook of Bilio-Pancreatic Diseases*, Piccin Nuova Libraria, S.p.A. Padova, 1986, pp. 2820–2825).
4. Bishop, W.J. *Early History of Surgery*, Barnes Noble Books N.Y. 1960, pp 77–142.
5. Yannos S, Athanasios P, Christos C, Evangelos F., History of biliary surgery. World J Surg. 2013;37(5):1006–1012. https://doi.org/10.1007/s00268-013-1960-6.
6. Longmire, WP Historic Landmarks in Biliary Surgery.pdf. South Med J. 1982; 75(12): 1548–1550.
7. Glenn F, Grafe WR. Historical Events in Biliary Tract Surgery. Arch Surg. 1966; 93(5): 848–852. https://doi.org/10.1001/archsurg.1966.01330050152025.
8. Ibid.
9. Ibid.
10. Praderi RC, Hess, W.A. Brief History of Biliopancreatic Diseases and Their Treatment, Part XII, in: Hess and Berci, *Textbook of Bilio-Pancreatic Diseases*, Piccin Nuova Libraria, S.p.A. Padova, 1986, pp. 2820–2825).
11. Yannos S, Athanasios P, Christos C, Evangelos F. History of biliary surgery. World J Surg. 2013;37(5):1006–1012. https://doi.org/10.1007/s00268-013-1960-6.
12. Ibid.
13. Glenn F, Grafe WR. Historical Events in Biliary Tract Surgery. Arch Surg. 1966; 93(5): 848–852. https://doi.org/10.1001/archsurg.1966.01330050152025.
14. Ibid.

Professor Dr. Hans Kehr (1862–1916)

Abstract

In 1888, Kehr received education in Vienna under Theodor Billroth and then in Berlin. He settled in surgical practice in Halberstadt, where he established a private surgical clinic and performed his first cholecystectomy in 1890. One of Kehr's attributes was a penchant for meticulous record keeping in addition to lecturing and publishing. His major contribution was his systematic approach and the pictorial illustrations that were created in the operating room. This translation of Kehr's *magnum opus* dealing with his own experience with cholecystectomy will hopefully preserve his name and assure that he is listed along with other giants who contributed to the principles of biliary surgery.

Keywords

Hans Kehr · Cholecystectomy · Surgical history Medical illustration

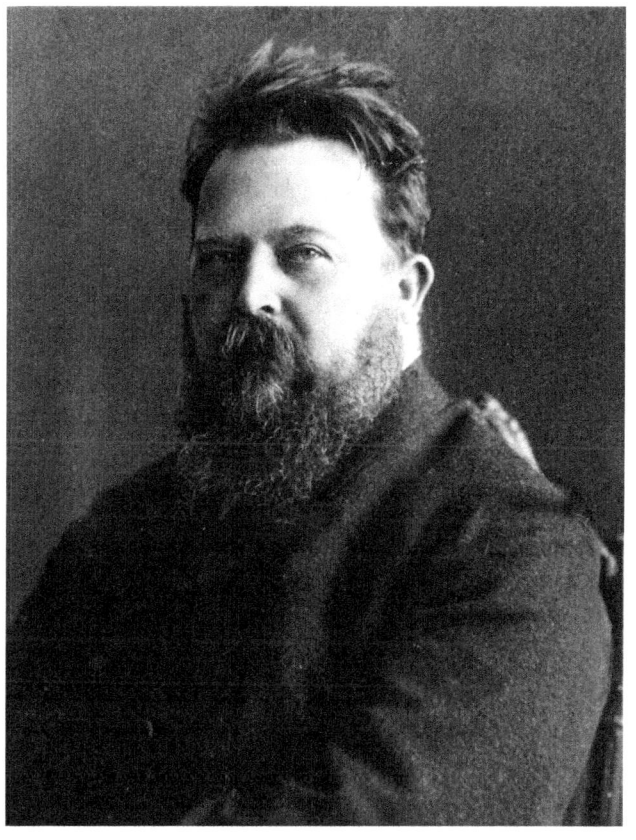

The best battle against infectious cholelithiasis is the surgeon's knife. – Hans Kehr

Hans Kehr (1862–1916) was the fifth of ten children born to Christophe Karl and Rosina Pauline Kehr [1]. His father was a distinct pedagogue whose precepts Kehr followed throughout life. Kehr studied in Jena, Halle and Berlin, obtaining his doctorate at Jena in 1884. After passing the state examination in Jena in 1885, he was assistant at the private surgical clinic of Ernst Meusel (1843–1914) in Gotha for 2 years.

In 1888, Kehr received further education in Vienna under Theodor Billroth (1829–1894) and then in Berlin. That same year he settled in surgical practice in Halberstadt, where he established a private surgical clinic. It was here that he performed his first cholecystectomy in 1890 on an indigent patient. His intense interest in biliary surgery led to a burgeoning practice which in a relatively short time achieved worldwide fame. Because of earlier success, Kehr was invited to take the chairmanship in Berlin and, from 1890 to 1916, published his experience in two volumes of 500 pages each (Published by Lehmann, Munich in 1913). During these 24 years he performed more than 2600 operations on the biliary system. Mayo and Halsted, famous American surgeons, also visited Kehr during this period.

One of Kehr's attributes was a penchant for meticulous record keeping in addition to lecturing and publishing [2]. By 1907, 10% of his patients were referrals from all parts of the world. Due to his pioneering work, he was appointed professor on the occasion of the 25th anniversary of the German Society of Surgery in 1897. In 1903, he was invited to the United States to lecture and to provide demonstrations in biliary surgery which greatly impressed his American surgical colleagues. In 1904, he was summoned to Paris to consult on the case of the prime minister of France, Pierre Marie Waldech-Rousseau (1846–1904).

In 1910, Kehr was appointed Privy Counsellor and moved to Berlin in order to concentrate his efforts entirely on biliary surgery. During this time, he pursued his interests in literature, music, and the arts. Kehr died of septicemia following injury to his finger during surgery [3].

For many years Kehr employed an artist, Mr. Frohse, who created drawings of his operative procedures. These illustrations, drawn more than 100 years ago, compete favorably with today's high-resolution photographic reproductions. Kehr was able to convince Mr. Frohse to stand behind him during every operation over many years to witness the dissections and make his drawings. In the evening hours, the two would discuss and improve the surgical illustrations.

They were able to produce a vast amount of data as well as the color documentation (see enclosures).

We selected this surgical pioneer because he was a meticulous and a superbly organized surgeon who established a patient recording system that included clinical history, examination, surgical procedures, and follow-up. His major contribution was this systematic approach and especially the pictorial illustrations that were created.

Kehr was also very interested in establishing a training system for residents, emphasizing the trainees need to know more about the details of anesthesia, still a relatively new concept in the late nineteenth century. Kehr was the first to put forth caveats about the use of chloroform in jaundiced patients because of its toxic effects on the impaired liver. He was also interested in operating room (OR) discipline; after 20 minutes of scrubbing, the anesthetic should not be initiated before the surgeon has the opportunity to talk with the patient. Anesthesia was performed in an adjacent room and the patient was transferred to the OR. In addition, the scrub nurse had to report that all instruments and other items for surgery were checked prior to the procedure and were available in the OR.

This translation of Kehr's *magnum opus* dealing with his own experience with cholecystectomy will hopefully preserve his name and assure that he is listed along with other giants who contributed to the principles of biliary surgery.

Summary of 25-pages Introduction by Professor Dr. Hans Kehr:

> I started working in a clinic in the small, German city of Halberstadt. The publisher (Lehmann) introduced me to an artist and painter, Mr. Frohse, who was with me for years and first learned the surgical environment, behavior, the patterns observed and my explanation of the surgery cases. I built for him a podium so that he could step up and observe surgery from a close distance and have an unobstructed view.
>
> Generally, he did the drawings in the morning, the coloring in the afternoon and we were able in the evenings to discuss the drawings, make corrections and interpretations. That was the reason that we started the illustrations in 1905. After seven years, we moved over to Berlin. He had a great sense of humor and mentioned that after observing 150 cases, he could make the surgery himself.
>
> In total, he was able to complete over 300 studies and a huge number of cases and giving me, for instance, the recommendation that in case of cystic artery bleeding during dissection, how I should take another finger, e.g., the left little finger to compress and prepare the suturing with an improved technique. This introduction was written in 1913. I remember well my first cholecystectomy in 1890.
>
> I was a follower of the famous German, Richard Wagner, to whose compositions I listened with great admiration. In my opinion, Wagner was also important to my father and my co-workers.
>
> The performance of the operation can be compared with a well-trained artist. The picture follows with a description of various explanations between a history and findings similar to music. Great agreement with Kocher's philosophy was described in great detail.

Kehr equates the performance of the operation with that of a well-trained artist or musician.

Kehr described memories of his father, who was a teacher and writer who published a book about the practice of teaching and learning in an elementary school translated into several languages. From this book, the younger Kehr made several citations.

Kehr explains that, "His writing and thinking were great symbols for my future." Kehr described in a page, the philosophy of his way of thinking in the performance of his father's teaching. He also described in great detail the style and the atmosphere of the operating rooms and Kehr made several citations from his father's publications. He expressed in detail the differences between practice and theory. Kehr described the importance of teaching truths at all times regarding his surgical outcomes.

Already in his introduction, he quoted the importance of the incision and the method of exploration and wound closure. He mentioned the importance of taking an accurate history from the patient and also quoted his philosophy that, "Art should stay art," as described by Goethe. He mentioned in great detail the theory of "not giving too much on the first sessions" and to be careful in using the word "experience."

Kehr included in his introduction that although he had performed more than 2600 cholecystectomies, he still believed that, "I am a beginner and need more experience."

In the next part of his introduction, he explains how important it is to create a precise patient history and how crucial it is in the learning period and general practice for a surgeon not to concentrate on the practical areas of surgery only. Kehr recommended that one pay attention to the patient's history and complete it with the appropriate questions as well as the postoperative instructions.

The first volume is written not only for surgeons, but also for internists. In the second volume, Kehr states that he "tried to describe the need to listen to the patient, the special operative technique as well as the post-operative treatment modalities." Kehr mentioned that it took his artist, Frohse, observations of 150 surgical procedures before he was able to start illustrating his case studies.

Frohse collaborated on 300 or more case studies and many post-mortem specimens. He predicted that a properly prepared and performed follow-up surgery was really an art. He expressed in great detail the cooperation of other colleagues who referred over 100 patients to his practice during the years. He alluded to the work of the famous pathologist, Ludwig Aschoff (1866–1942), was important in the area of pancreas problems.

Special attention was given to his scrub nurse and other nurses and personnel involved in patient care. He mentioned also the reproduction of colorful pictures to be of significant help in the descriptions of findings.

This is a very detailed personalized introduction which is unique in style. It is also a detailed philosophy of Kehr's approach to surgery and medicine which included references to art and music.

References

1. Morgenstern L. Hans Kehr: not first, but foremost. Surg Endosc, 1993;7:152–154.
2. Ibid.
3. Ibid.

Translation of Professor Dr. Hans Kehr

Practice of Biliary Surgery

Descriptions and Pictures of Professor Dr. H. Kehr

Volume 1

Munich

JF Lehmann, Publisher

1913

Die Chirurgie in Einzeldarstellungen

herausgegeben von Prof. Dr. R. Grashey

Bd. I

Die Praxis der Gallenwege-Chirurgie

von

Prof. Dr. H. Kehr

Bd. I

München
J. F. Lehmann's Verlag

Surgery of Single Cases
Presented by Professor R. Grashey, Munich
Volume I and II

The Practice of Biliary Surgery

Two Volumes for Internists and Surgeons by

Professor Dr. Hans Kehr

Volume I:

Preparation for Surgery of the Biliary System General Technique of Surgery

Volume II:

Special Technique of Biliary Surgery And

Post-operative Treatment and Results

Munich

J. F. Lehmann Publisher

1913

DIE CHIRURGIE IN EINZELDARSTELLUNGEN.

Herausgegeben von Professor Dr. Rudolf Grashey in München.

I. u. II. Band.

Die

Praxis der Gallenwege-Chirurgie
in Wort und Bild.

Ein Atlas und Lehrbuch in 2 Bänden
für Interne und Chirurgen.

Auf Grund eigener, bei 2000 Laparotomien gesammelter Erfahrungen bearbeitet

von

Professor Dr. Hans Kehr

Geh. Sanitätsrat in Berlin.

Erster Band:
Die Vorbereitungen zu einer Operation an den Gallenwegen und die allgemeine Technik der Gallenwege-Chirurgie.

Zweiter Band:
Die spezielle Technik der Gallenwege-Chirurgie mit Einschluss der Nachbehandlung und der Operationserfolge.

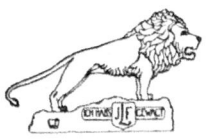

MÜNCHEN
J. F. LEHMANN'S VERLAG
1913.

Contents of Volume I

	Page
INTRODUCTION	7
Index of Tables	28
Catalogue of Illustrations	30

Part I

I.	Introduction	3
II.	Preparation of Surgery	
	1. Instruments	16
	2. The Patient	27
	3. The Surgeon and Assistant	35

Part II

I.	The Normal Anatomy of the Biliary System	
	1. The anatomy of the biliary tract	43
	2. The nerves and lymphatic vessels of the biliary tract	111
	3. The abnormalities of the biliary tract, art, hepatica and cystica	115
II.	Some Remarks on the Physiology of Bile	153
III.	The Pathological Anatomy of Cholelithiasis	157
IV.	The Symptomatology and Diagnosis of Cholelithiasis	209
V.	The prognosis and the internal treatment of cholelithiasis	272
VI.	About the indications for internal and surgical treatment of cholelithiasis	297

Part III.

I.	Anesthesia	345
II.	Positioning of the patient and surgical staff	349
III.	Abdominal wall incision	354
IV.	Sterility during surgery	366
V.	Adhesions	370
VI.	Suturing of skin incision	376
VII.	Short Summary of Surgical Procedure	392
	Epilogue	401
	Authors and Contributions	405
	Alphabetic Register	406

Inhaltsverzeichnis des I. Bandes.

	Seite
Vorwort	VII
Verzeichnis der Tafeln	XXVIII
Verzeichnis der Textabbildungen	XXX

I. Teil.

I. Einleitende Bemerkungen	3
II. Die Vorbereitungen zu einer Gallensteinoperation.	
1. Die Vorbereitungen der Instrumente, des Verbandmaterials, der Seide etc.	16
2. Die Vorbereitungen des Kranken	27
3. Die Vorbereitungen des Arztes und seiner Assistenten	35

II. Teil.

I. Die normale Anatomie des Gallensystems.	
1. Die Anatomie der Gallenwege. (Gallenblase, D. cysticus und D. choledocho-hepaticus.)	43
2. Die Nerven und Lymphgefässe der Gallenwege	111
3. Die Anomalien der Gallenwege, der art. hepatica und cystica	115
II. Einige Bemerkungen zur Physiologie der Galle	153
III. Die pathologische Anatomie der Cholelithiasis	157
IV. Die Symptomatologie und Diagnostik der Cholelithiasis	209
V. Die Prognose und die interne Behandlung der Cholelithiasis	272
VI. Ueber die Indikationen zur internen und chirurgischen Behandlung der Cholelithiasis	297

III. Teil.

I. Die Narkose bei einer Operation an den Gallenwegen	345
II. Lagerung des Kranken, Verteilung der bei einer Operation an den Gallenwegen beschäftigten Personen	349
III. Die Bauchwandschnitte bei einer Operation an den Gallenwegen	354
IV. Die Asepsis während einer Gallensteinoperation	366
V. Die Lösung der Verwachsungen bei einer Gallensteinoperation	370
VI. Ueber die Tamponade und die Naht der Bauchwunde nach einer Gallensteinoperation	376
VII. Kurze Uebersicht über die Operationsmethoden an den Gallenwegen. Die Verteilung der Steine in den Gallengängen und ihr Nachweis bei geöffneter Bauchhöhle	392
Nachwort	401
Autoren- und Namen-Register	405
Alphabetisches Sachregister	408

Instruments

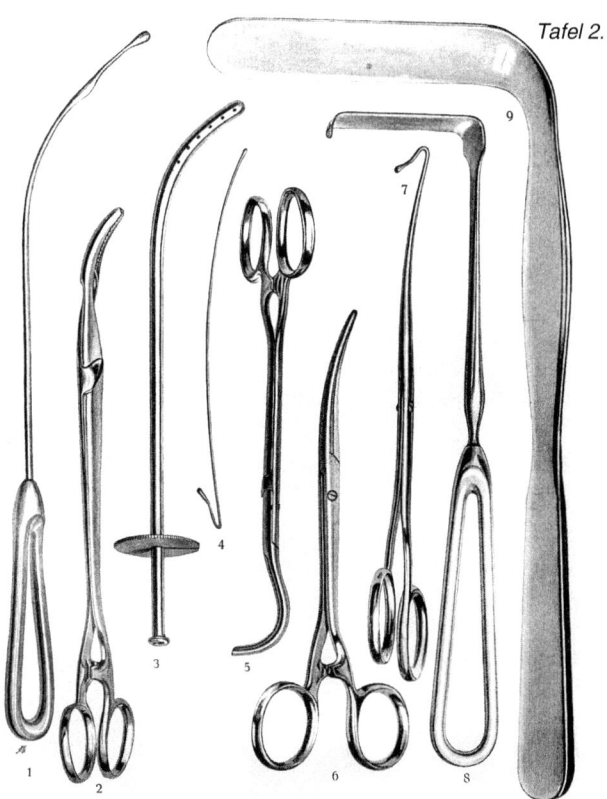

Tafel 2.

Retractors for Biliary Surgery

Kehr was keen to have the tools available in a sterile form and that the resident and nurse were aware of their proper presentation.

He also identified the instrument name:

1. Uterus or papilla duodenal probe
2. Mikulicz forceps
3. Irrigation – suction tube from Ultzman
4. Malleable probe
5, 6. Curved forceps after Pean
7. Small probe with miniature jaws
8. Langenbuch's retractor
9. Large retractor from Martin

Kehr was keen to give credit to the originator or designer. The resident scrubbing with him had to learn and use carefully the well-designed tools. Kehr used, in every cholecystectomized patient, a soft or malleable probe to introduce through the transected cystic duct to probe the CBD and get a feel about stones. He repeated this also in the hepatic ducts (replaced later by Choledochoscopy).

Instruments

Original idea, designed a century ago to have T-tube drainage avoiding postoperative bile leakage and/or peritonitis.

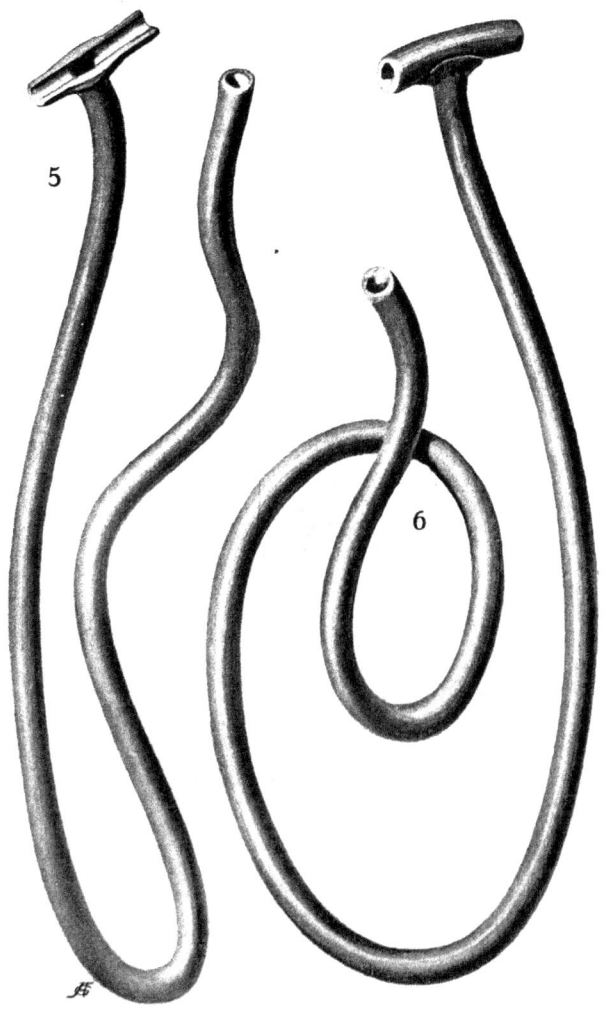

T-Tubes
Designed by Kehr and made in different (3) diameters for draining the choledochus or the use of straight tubes to drain dilated ducts.

In case of retained stones and a drained CBD: 2 weeks of repeated irrigation attempting to move the stone into the duodenum after a more relaxed sphincter. These patients were followed in the postoperative period for months (including repeated irrigations).

Description of Surgical Cases (Bilingual) Translation

Case 48
  Table 39
  38-year-old female from Gustrow
  Admission: May 24, 1905
  Surgery: May 25, 1905
  Discharge: June 30, 1906. Cured
  Two-year history of severe pain at right side of abdomen. No icterus. No fever.
  Surgery: Small gallbladder, severe adhesions at the fundus, thick edematous wall, midsize stone in gallbladder.
  OR Time: 20 minutes
  Histology: Chronic inflammation. No cancer.
Figure 2: Very small gallbladder with many scars.
  Diagnosis: Cholecystitis
  Surgery: Small gallbladder with one large stone. Ectomy. No postoperative complaints
  OR Time: 20 minutes

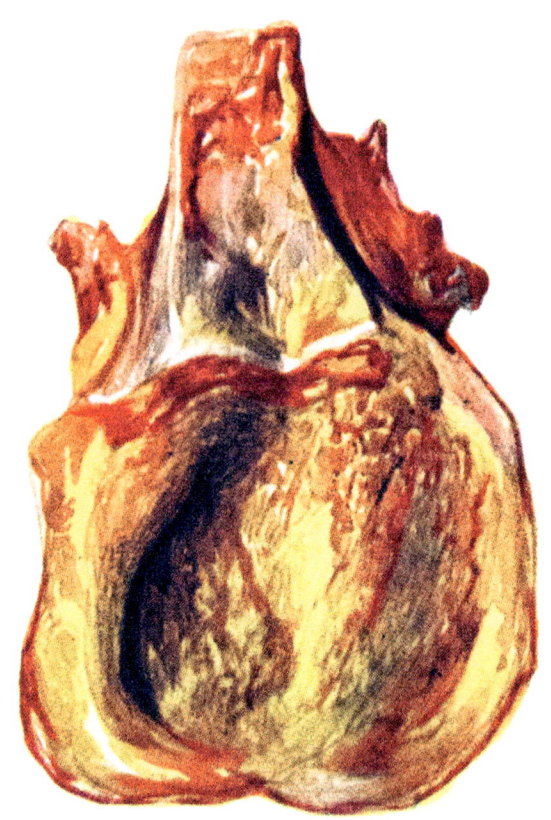

Fig. 2.
Kr.-G. Nr. 48.

Krankengeschichte Nr. 48 (Tafel 39, Fig. 2)
B.B.m 38 jähr. Kaufmannsfrau aus Gűstrow,
Aufgen.: 24.5.1905.
Operiert: 25.5.1905. Ektomie.
Entlassen: 30.6.1905. Geheilt.
Anamnese: Im Jahre 1894 nacths zum erstenmal ein Magenkrampfanfall (7 gedruckte Zeilen).

Befund: Lieber nicht vergrössert, kein Tumor der Gallenblasse palpable, doch grosse Schmertzhaftigkeit bei calculosa.

Diagnose: Cholecystitis chronica calculosa.

Operation: 25.5.05. Gallenblase klein mit grossen Solitärstein.

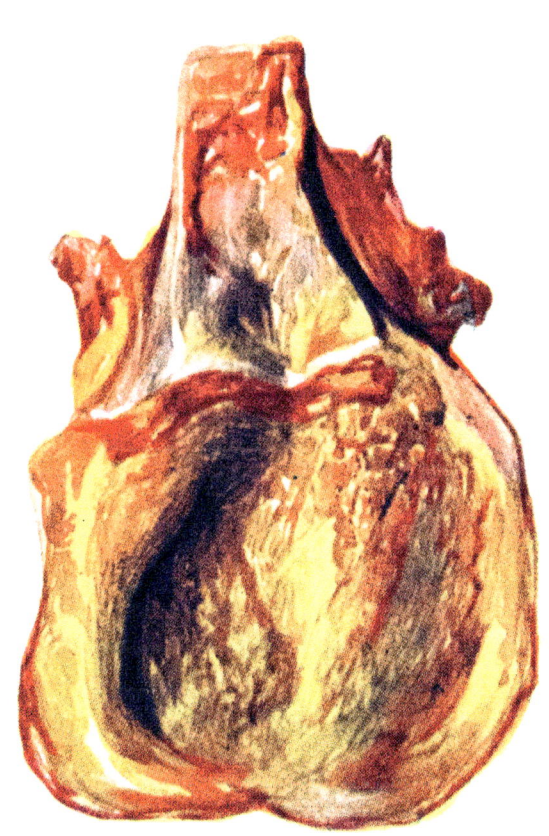

Fig. 2.
Kr.-G. Nr. 48.

Summarized Translation

Case: 53
Table 40
44-year-old male teacher from Langenstein.

Admission: May 3, 1905
Surgery: May 7, 1905
Discharge: May 8, 1905. Mortality

Cholecystectomy, drainage of CBD and Hepatic Duct. Duodenal injuries. History: 2 years of severe right subcostal pain. Loss of 30 lbs. weight.

Findings, Right subcostal tenderness, no icterus. Developed severe pain requiring morphium.

Diagnosis: Chronic Cholecystitis.

Surgery: Thick gallbladder. Aspirations, Gallstones removed during dissection of gallbladder. During difficult dissections with multiple duodenal injuries and repair were made. Dilated CBD with 15 stones. Drainage.

Injury of artery with severe bleeding, difficulties repair. OR Time: 1 hour, 15 minutes.

4 weeks later sudden death (cardiac?)

History Chronic inflammation of Gallbladder (Summary)

(See opposite page for size of detailed report.)

Krankengeschichte Nr. 53 (Tafel 40, Fig. 2). ...

W. A., 44 jähr. Hauptlehrer aus Langenstein.

Aufgen.: 3. 5. 1905.

Operiert: 7. 5. 1905. Ektomie. Hepatikusdrainage. Choledochusdrainage. Hepatopexie. Uebernähung von Duodenaldefekten.

Entlassen: 8. 5. 1905. Exitus.

Anamnese: August 1903 akut einsetzender Choledochusverschluss. Fast 2 Jahre ging es dem Patienten gut, bis vor 5 Wochen nachts wieder Gallensteinkolik eintrat. Vor 3 Wochen besonders starke Schmerzen. Infolge der geringen Nahrungsaufnahme in der letzten Zeit ziemlich an Gewicht abgenommen, einige 30 Pfund.

Befund: Sehr anämisch aussehender Mann, in der Gallenblasengegend geringe Resistenz, keine Schmerzhaftigkeit.

Verlauf: 4. 5. Gegen Mittag plötzlich starke Kolik, die eine Morphiuminjektion nötig macht. In der Nacht vom 6. 5. zum 7. 5. wieder Kolik, kein Gallenfarbstoff im Urin, dieser ganz hell.

Diagnose: Chronische Cholecystitis (Steine im Choledochus?). Ulcus duodeni nicht völlig auszuschliessen.

Operation: 7. 5. Wellenschnitt. Leber etwas vergrössert, sehr weich. Gallenblase verdickt, entzündet, langgestreckt, enthält sehr wenig Flüssigkeit und kleine Steine. Aspiration von trüber Galle, Gallenblase flächenhaft mit Duodenum verwachsen. Dieses zeigt im mittleren Teil eine narbige harte Stelle (ausgeheiltes Ulcus duodeni). Bei der Loslösung reisst das Duodenum an 2 Stellen ein. Sorgfältige Naht. Choledochus sehr erweitert, enthält kleine Steine. Ektomie der Gallenblase, sowie des Cystikus. Cysticotomie. Choledochotomie. Im stark erweiterten Hepatikus und Choledochus Steine, im Hepatikus 3, im Choledochus 15, mehrere retroduodenal. Rohr in den Hepatikus und Rohr in den Choledochus. Bei der wasserdichten Vernähung der Choledochusinzision wird eine starke Arterie angestochen. Sehr heftige Blutung, Unterbindung. 3 Tampons. Hepatopexie, doch ist die Leber so morsch, dass die Fäden durchschneiden; nur bei sehr lockerer Knotung gibt das Lebergewebe nicht nach. Dauer der Operation $5/4$ Stunden. Die chronisch entzündete Gallenblase zeigt im Fundus Ulcerationen, am Hals ist die Drüse geschwollen, der Cystikus ist stark erweitert. In der Gallenblase ca. 40 erbsengrosse Steine.

Verlauf: Tod am 8. 5. 05 an Herzschwäche.

Die mikroskopische Untersuchung der Gallenblase in Marburg ergab folgendes:

Mikroskopisch erwiesen sich die Schleimhautzotten leicht papillenartig verdickt. Das Epithel senkt sich stellenweise divertikelartig durch die Muskularis hindurch fast bis an die Serosa. Schleimdrüsen wurden vermisst. In der Subserosa der verdickten Serosa fand sich eine beträchtliche, durch rundzellige und eosinophilgekörnte Leukocyten bedingte Infiltration. Diese erstreckt sich ein Ende weit, entlang den Lymphspalten, in die Muskularis. Die in der Serosa vorhandenen Gefässe sind dickwandig.

Epikrise: Patient sollte schon Mitte April zur Operation kommen, doch hatte er zu grosse Angst vor derselben; da er die letzten 6 Wochen fast gar nichts ass, war er sehr geschwächt. Der Tod ist auf Herzschwäche und Lungenödem zurückzuführen. Der blasse anämische, früher recht korpulente, jetzt sehr abgemagerte Mann konnte den schweren $5/4$ stündigen Eingriff nicht überwinden. Am Operationsgebiet war alles in Ordnung; die Leber war bereits mit dem Peritoneum parietale verklebt (20 St. post op.); keine Nachblutung. Wunde sauber, Rohre lagen gut. Eine Sektion des Herzens war nicht möglich.

Summarized Translation

Case 2

W.S., a 45-year old builder from Namslau Admission: 11-10-1912
Surgery: 11-12-1912, Ectomy
Discharge: 3-11-1913, Cured

For 10 months, severe painful abdominal attacks at right upper quadrant position of abdomen. Dark urine recently. Loss of weight (25 lbs.).

Surgery: Large gallbladder with multiple adhesions to the surrounding tissues. Large stone impacted at the upper part of cystic duct (See Figure2).

Duration of Surgery: 35 minutes Discharged free of symptoms.

Krankengeschichte Nr. 2.

W. S., 45 jähr. Braumeister aus Namslau.

Aufgen.: 16.8.1912. Wieder aufgen.: 10.11.1912.
Operiert: 12.11.1912. Ektomie.
Entlassen: 30.11.1912. Geheilt.

Anamnese: Im Januar 1912 erster schwerer Anfall mit Schmerzen rechts im Oberbauch. Dauer des Anfalls 4 Stunden. Fieber hat bestanden. Im Februar 1912 einige Anfälle. Im März drei Anfälle mit Fieber, manchmal war weisser Stuhlgang, dunkler Urin. Ende März ging Patient nach Karlsbad, wo er 4 Anfälle mit Fieber und Gelbsucht hatte. Zwei Wochen nach Karlsbad ein heftiger Anfall, welcher 2 Stunden anhielt, aber ohne Fieber. Dann folgten in unregelmässigen Zwischenräumen mehrere Anfälle, oft mit weissem Stuhlgang. Am 5. Juli sind Steine nach einer Oelkur abgegangen. Hinterher noch 5 Anfälle. An Körpergewicht hat P. in einem halben Jahre 25 Pfund verloren.

17.8.12. Patient verliess, wegen Anratens der Operation, die Klinik.

10.11.12. Nach Weggang aus der Klinik etwa alle 2 Tage, seit 14 Tage beinahe jeden Tag einen Anfall: ein einziges Mal 8 Tage beschwerdefrei.

Diagnose: Cholecystitis chronica. (Adhäsionen?)
Soziale Indikation.

Befund: Druckempfindliche Resistenz der Gallenblasengegend. Urin frei.

Operation: 12.11.11. Gallenblase gross, einige Verwachsungen mit Netz. Lösung. Sehr fettes lig. cystico-duodenale. (Fig. 2.) Im Hals ein Stein. Art. cystica muss in sehr grosser Tiefe unterbunden werden. Cysticus ganz eng und zart; da das Operationsfeld ausserordentlich tief liegt, wird auf Choledochusspaltung verzichtet. Der Stein ist zudem ein radiärer Cholesterinstein. Gallenblase war sehr verdickt. 2 Tampons.

Dauer der Operation: 35 Min.

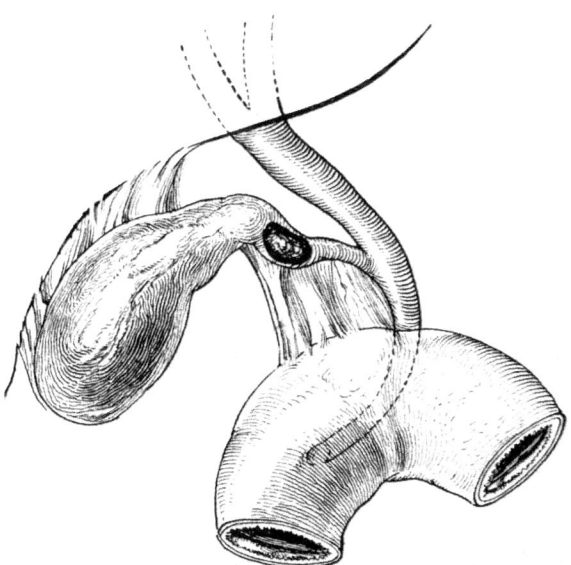

Fig. 2.
Lig. cystico-duodenale.

A stone position in cystic duct

The Anatomy and Variations of Important Structures

52

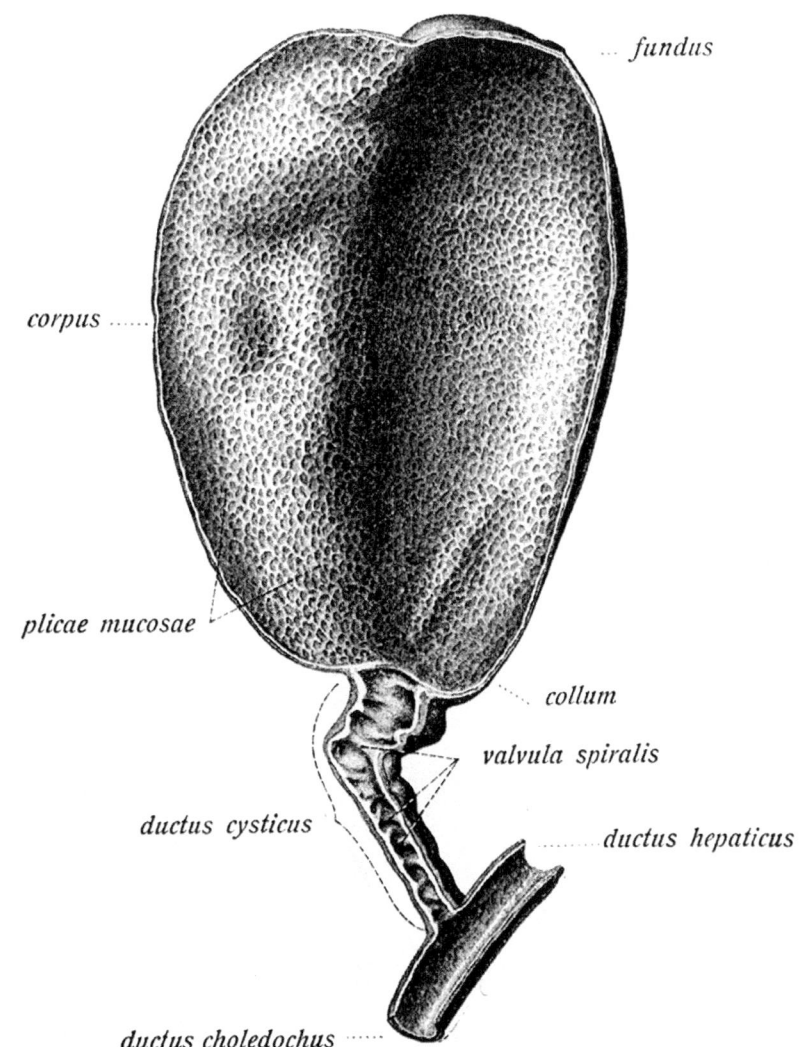

Die normale, d. h. durch Entzündung nicht erweiterte und verdickte Gallenblase hat die Form einer Birne und liegt zwischen lobus quadratus und dem rechten Leberlappen in der fossa vesicae felleae, die dem vorderen Abschnitt der fossa sagittalis dextra entspricht. Man unterscheidet an der Gallenblase (Figur 3) einen Fundus, ein Corpus und ein Collum. Die Länge einer normalen Gallenblase beträgt 7—9 cm und zeigt am Fundus einen Durchmesser von ca. 3 cm. Bei normaler Füllung der Gallenblase — ihre Kapazität dürfte 30—40 ccm betragen — überragt der Fundus gewöhnlich den vorderen scharfen Leberrand, welcher hier eine leichte Einbuchtung (incisura vesicalis) aufweist. Doch trifft man auch genug Gallenblasen, deren Fundus um einige Zentimeter höher steht als der Leberrand. Das ist fast regelmässig der Fall bei den durch Entzündung geschrumpften Gallenblasen; aber auch bei gesunden Gallenblasen kann man einen solchen Hochstand der Gallenblase recht oft feststellen. Man unterscheidet an der Gallenblase eine obere und untere Wandung. Die obere ist durch Bindegewebe mit der Leberkapsel verlötet. Die untere Wandung ist mit Peritoneum überzogen, welches links vom lobus quadratus, rechts vom rechten Leberlappen auf die Gallenblase übergeht.

Another sample of cystic duct configuration

erstellen kann.
:ndung ist sehr einfach. Man führt die Sonde ca. 2 cm tief
ıchus ein und zieht sie dann langsam zurück. (Fig. 8.) Ihr Haken
:r dem Sporn, den der
  D. hepaticus miteinan-
 . 9.) Ist man mit dem
  D. hepaticus, so zieht
e kräftig an und kann
)atikus-Eingang zugäng-
  dass nunmehr die Ein-
  oder Rinnenrohres ge-
  der Hepatikus-Eingang
ıg, so spaltet man den
  Sonde und stellt sich
ten Zugang zum D. he-
  dass nunmehr die Ein-
ˈohres leicht gelingt.
  den Krankengeschichten
gehen eingehender be-

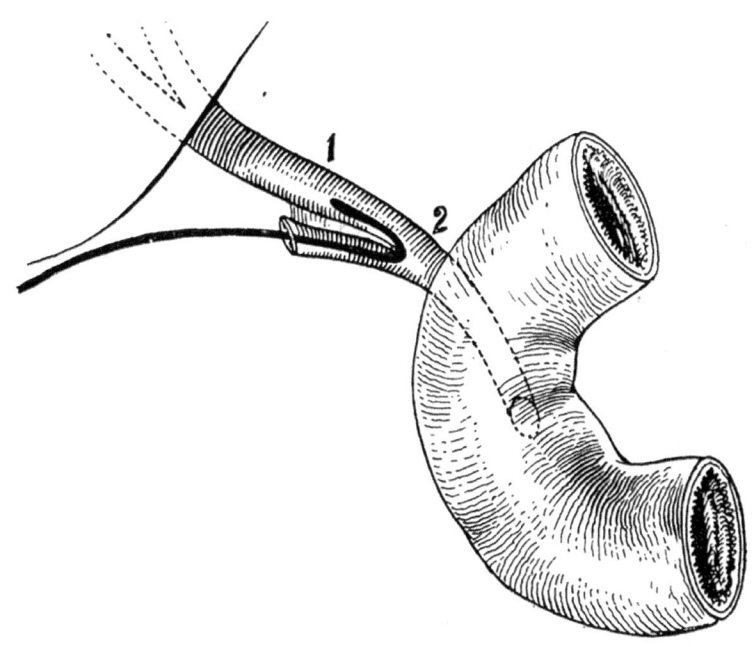

Die Angelsonde ist so zurückgezogen, dass sie den Sporn zwischen dem D. cysticus und D. hepaticus fängt. Spaltung des Sporns von 1 bis 2 (Hepaticotomia interna).

A malleable soft probe introduced through the cystic duct to the hepatic or distal duct to feel resistance (stone). Earlier ideas about choledochoscopy.

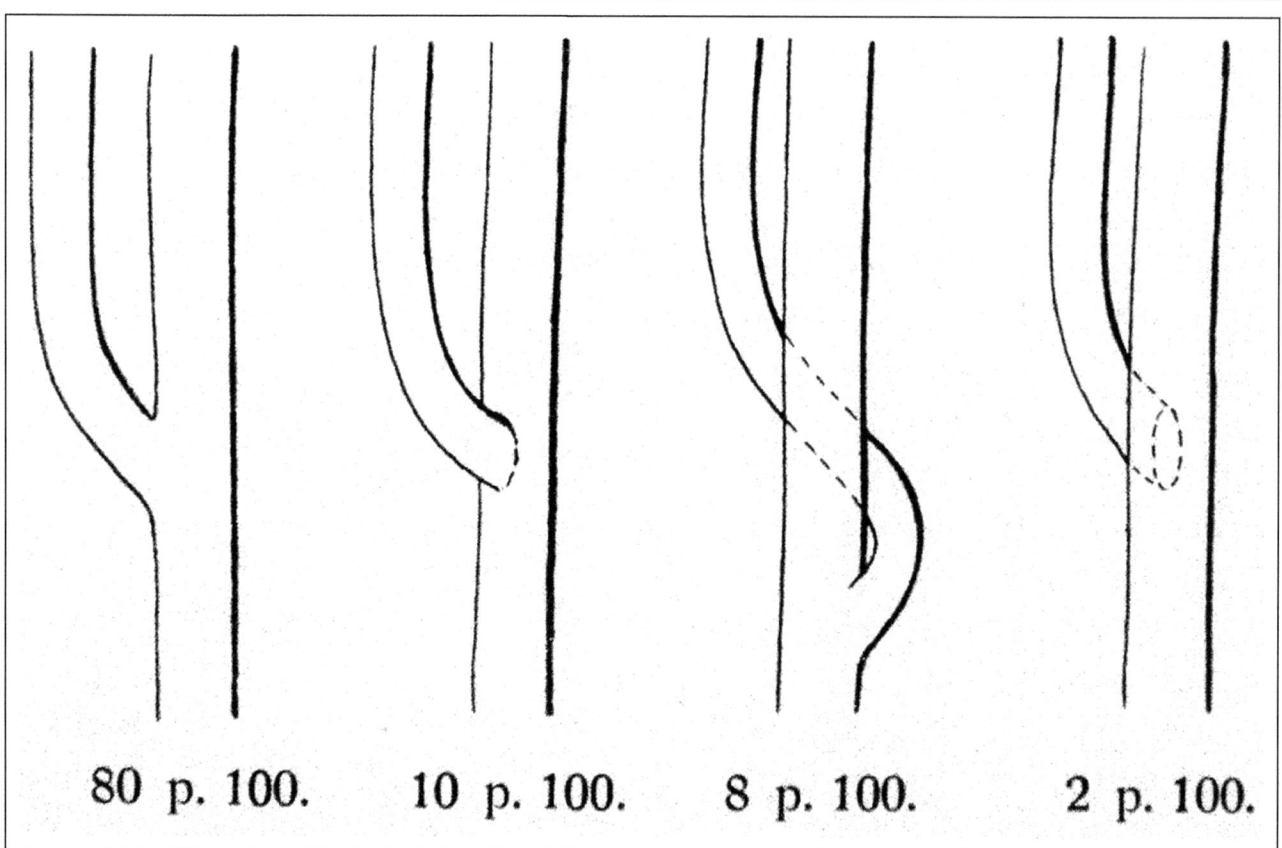

(Page 107) Attention was drawn 100 years ago about the anatomical variations of the cystic duct anatomy and various anomalies, and the importance of recognizing them during dissections.

4 The Anatomy and Variations of Important Structures

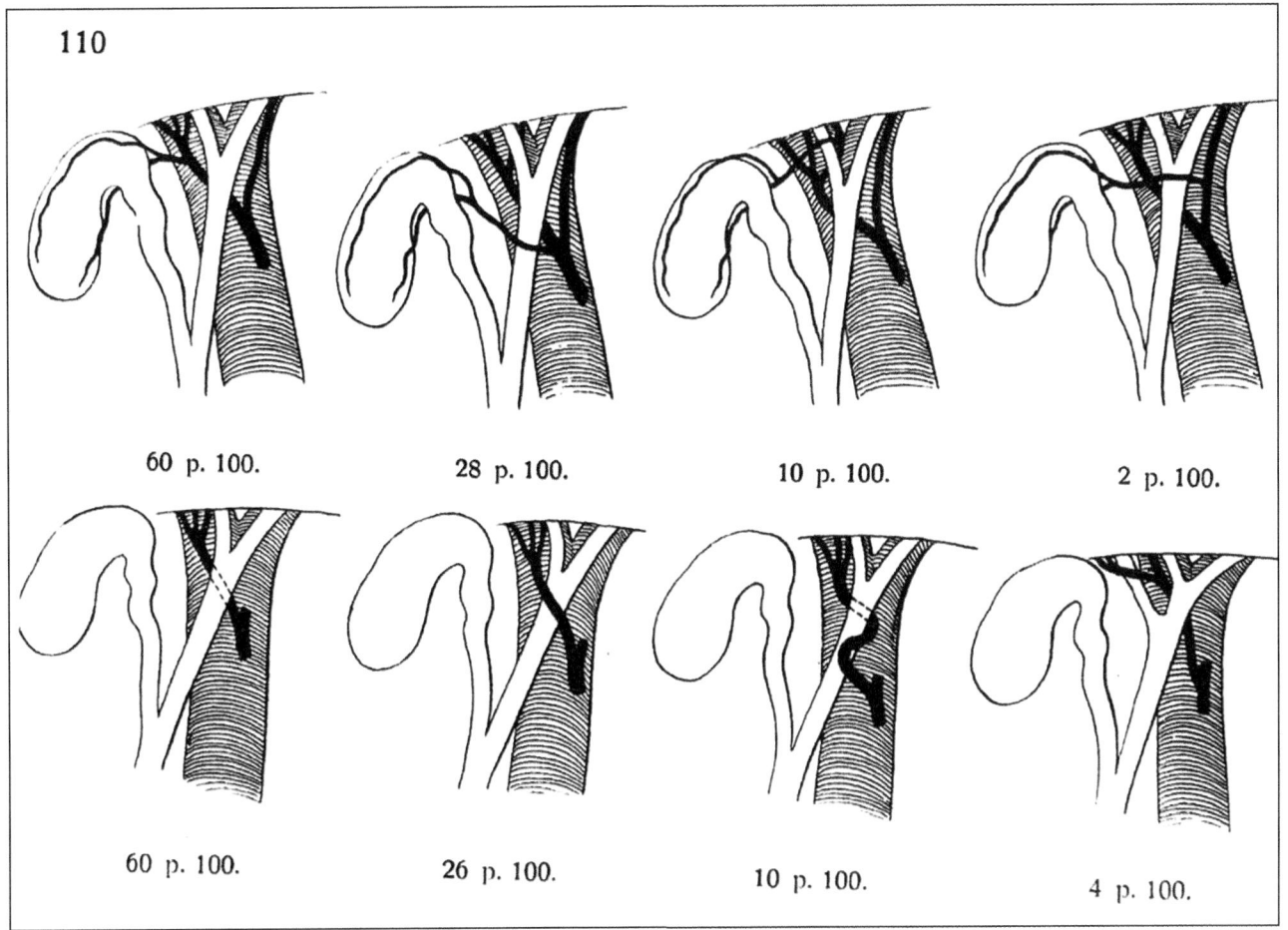

Two full pages of anatomical variations are described about cystic duct configurations

The top row, Figs. 51, 52, 53, and 54 show the configuration of the cystic artery and possibilities of injuries when anomalies occur.

Figures 55, 56, 57, and 58 display the right branch of the hepatic artery. Any changes of the anatomy can lead to severe bleeding.

Table 20

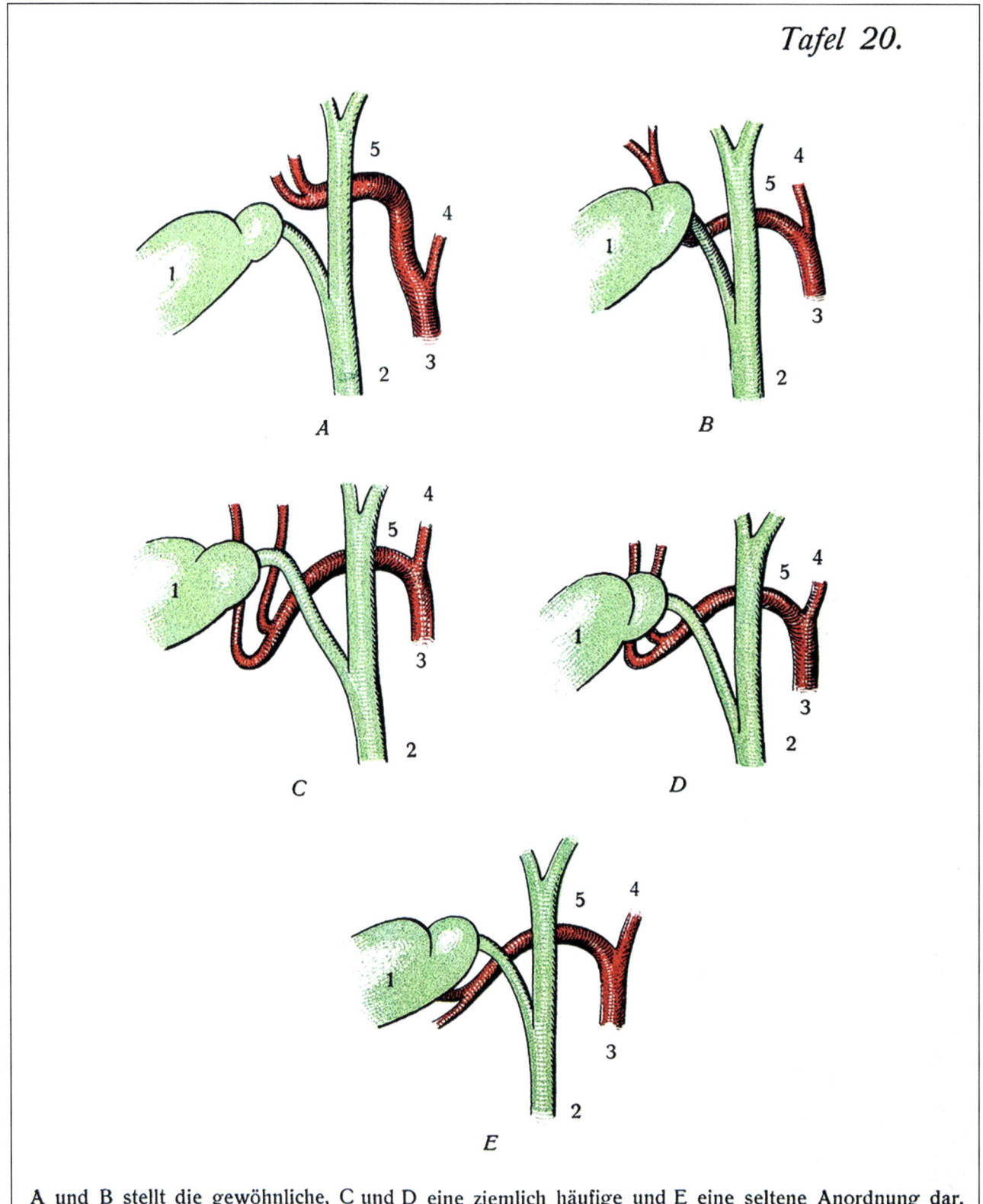

A und B stellt die gewöhnliche, C und D eine ziemlich häufige und E eine seltene Anordnung dar.
1 Gallenblase.
2 D. choledochus.
3 Art. hepatica propria.
4 Ramus sinister art. hepaticae.
5 Ramus dexter art. hepaticae.

Hepatic artery anatomy and variations (more details in book, pages 108–110)

Biliary Stones 5

Table 34

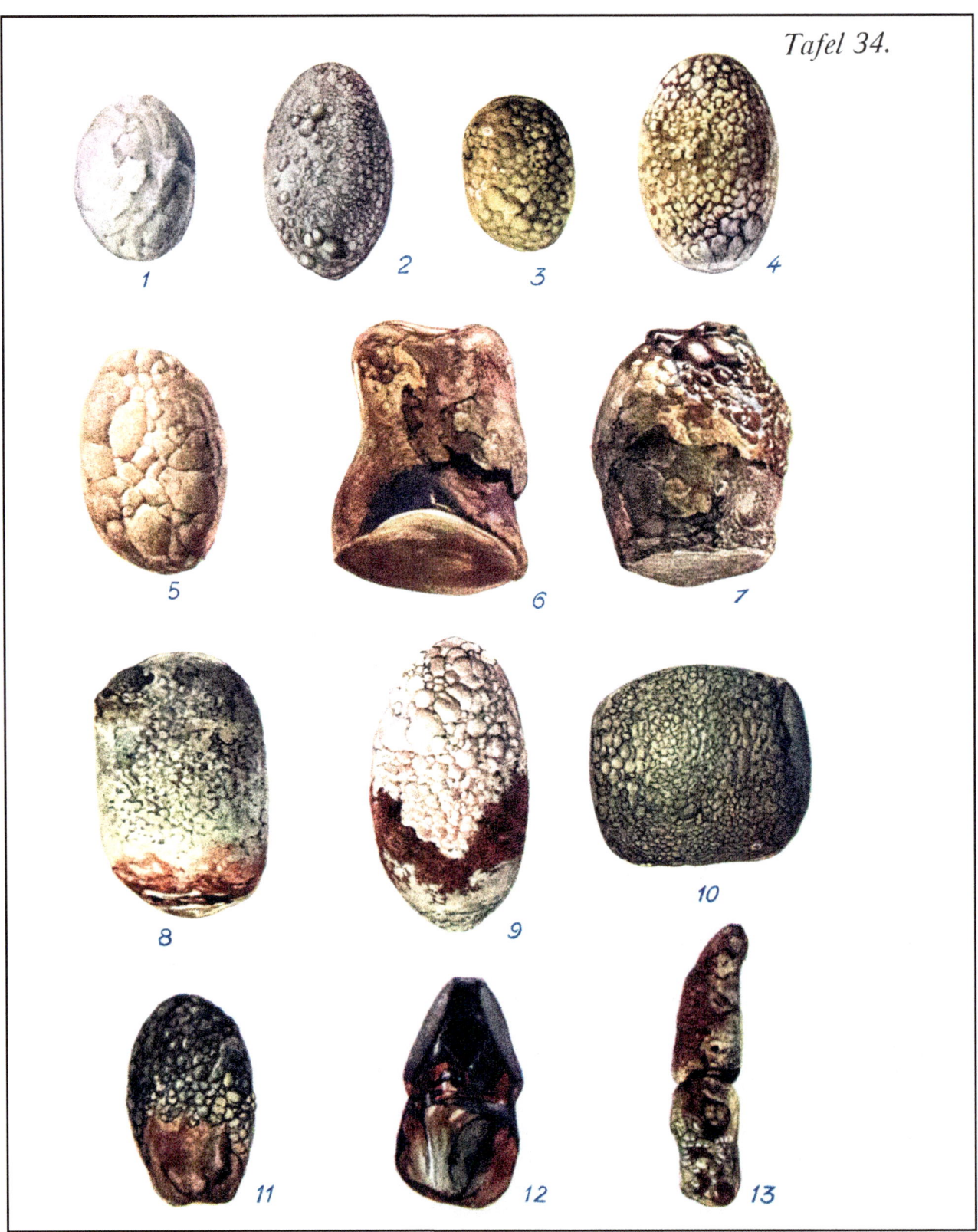

5 Biliary Stones

Calculi

Stones of actual sizes, calculi can be of bilirubin pigment, calcium composition.

No. 1: White cholesterol stones
No. 2, 3, 4: Thick calcium conglomerate
No. 5: Segmented stone
No. 6–7: Stones caused ileus in supraduodenal choledochus. No. 8: Stones with interesting surface
No. 13: Elongated soft calculus which took the shape or configuration of the choledochus.

Table 35

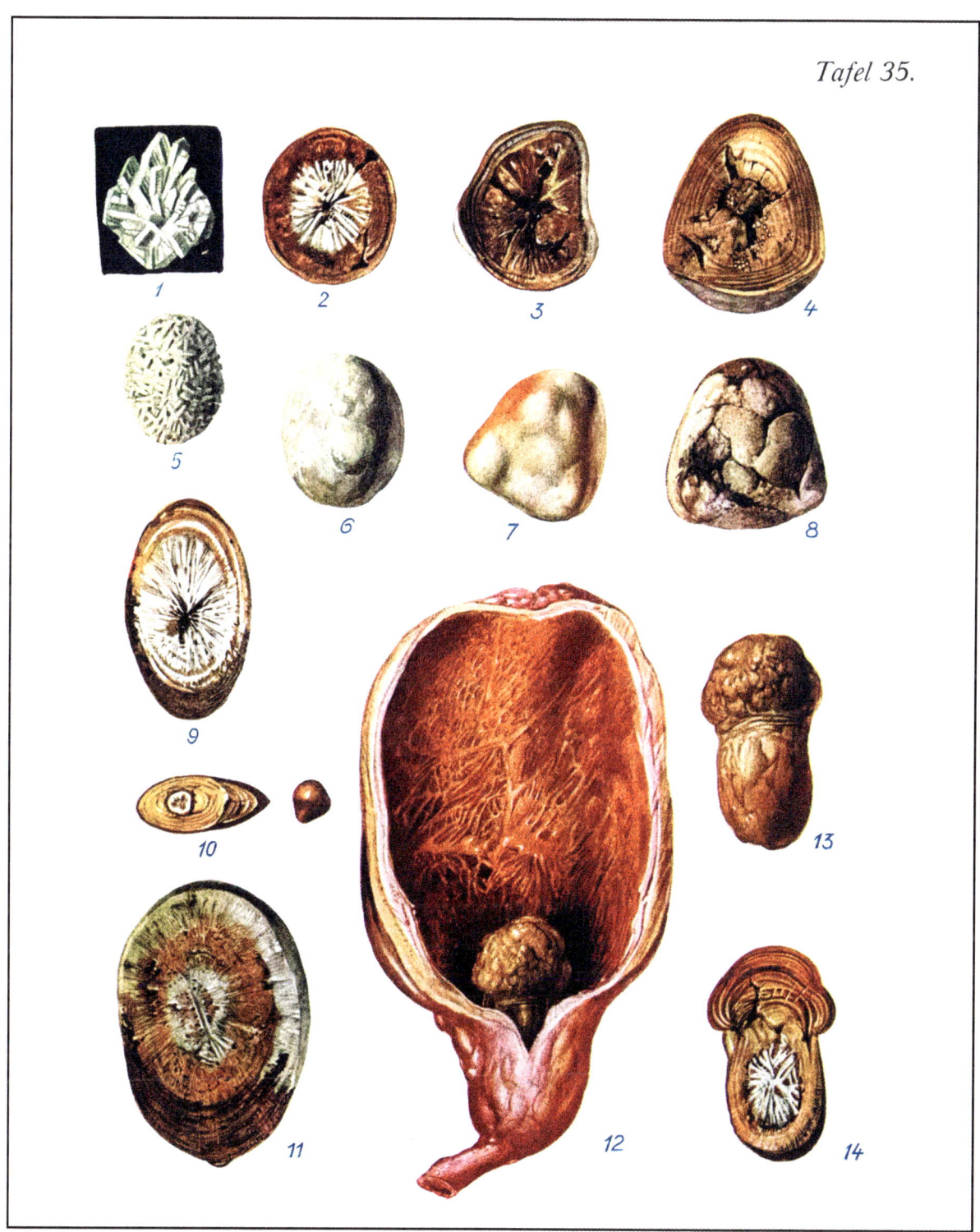

Tafel 35.

Calculi and Gallbladder

No. 1: It was found coincidentally in the gallbladder by surgery of carcinoma of the gallbladder.

Nos. 2–11 and 14–15 were found as a single calculus in a gallbladder (detailed description of stone composition on page 170 of Kehr's book and reference to Aschoff publication, *Cholelithiasis*).

No. 12: Gallbladder with characteristic appearance of the wall and stones.

Summarized Case Report

Case: 42
 Table 45
 65-year-old widow from Sandersleben
 Admitted: 5-23-1905
 Surgery: 5-24-1905
 Discharged: 7-15-1905, Cured

Summarized report: 7 years history of periodic pain in the mid-abdominal with radiation to the back. No jaundice.

Surgery: Distended hemorrhagic gallbladder with adhesions. Small cystic duct, cholecystectomy.

Duration of Surgery: 35 minutes (!)

Pathology: Severe hemorrhagic all partially necrotic gallbladder cystitis with severe hemorrhagic infarctions. No malignancy.

See Fig. 1.

Case: 43
Table 45
50-year-old female secretary and wife from Magdeberg
Admitted: 6-25-1905
Surgery: 6-29-1905
Died: 7-1-1905

2-year history of abdominal pain, jaundice, enlarged liver, dark urine.

Operation: Enlarged gallbladder, ascitic fluid, dilated common bile duct with a large palpable stone. Choledochotomy and t-tube drainage, enlarged pancreas and enlarged liver.

Duration of Surgery: 45 minutes

History: No malignancy, chronic ulcerative colitis. Severe bleeding from the wound, sudden death on 7-1-1905 (emboli?).

See Fig. 2.

Table 45

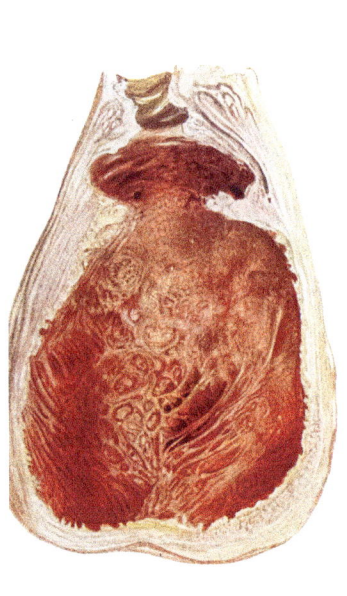
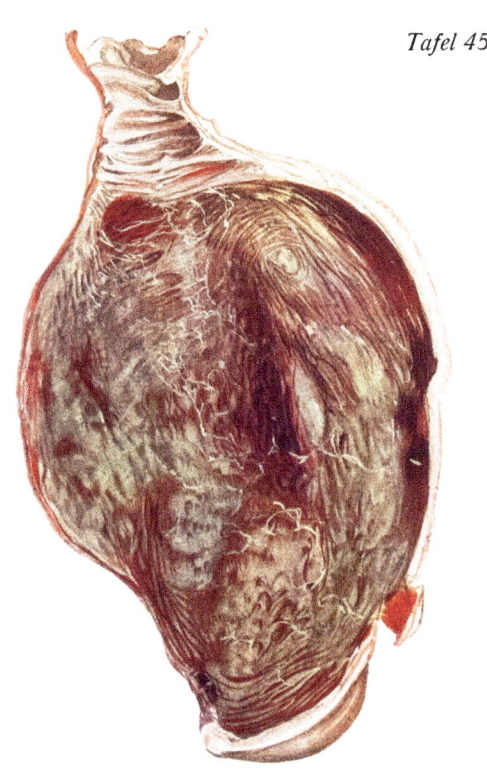

Tafel 45.

Case 44
Table 38
34-year-old female from Chernovitz
Admitted: June 20, 1905
Surgery: June 22, 1905
Discharged: October 22, 1905

Typical abdominal cramps. No jaundice, no fever. Tenderness in right upper quadrant.

Surgery: difficult case because of adhesions, distended gallbladder with multiple stones. Severe adhesions. Difficult ectomy because of bleeding.

Duration of Surgery: 1½ hours.

Histology: Chronic severe cholecystitis. No malignancy.

Postoperative: Venous thrombosis.

See **Fig. 1**: Hemorrhagic gallbladder with a large stone.

Case 45
Table 38
38-year-old woman from Haberstadt
Admitted: 6-23-1905
Surgery: 6-25-1905
Discharge: 7-17-1905, Cured

For 2 weeks, surgeries repeated right subcostal painful colic. No jaundice.

Chronic cholecystitis.

Surgery: Adhesions. Gallbladder removed. Common bile duct looked normal size.

Duration of Surgery: 25 minutes.

Histology: Empyema of gallbladder with adhesions.

See **Fig. 2**.

Summarized Case Report

Case 46
Table 38
36-year-old female teacher from Remscheid
Admission: 7-5-1905
Surgery: 7-7-1905
Discharge: 7-17-1905

History of 3 years of colicky pain right subcostal area loss of weight. Very nervous patient, right subcostal tenderness, clear urine. No jaundice.

Surgery: Many adhesions, appendectomy, hemorrhagic gallbladder, slightly distended with a palpable stone. Operative time: 30 minutes.

See **Fig. 3**.

Table 38

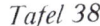

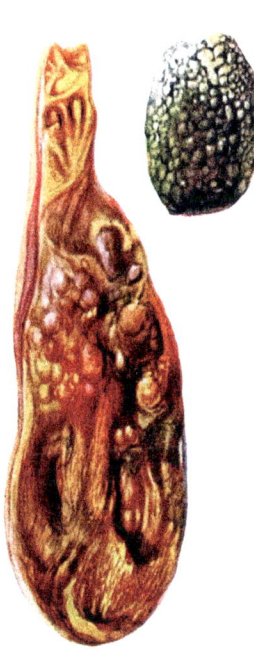

Kr.-G. Nr. 44.

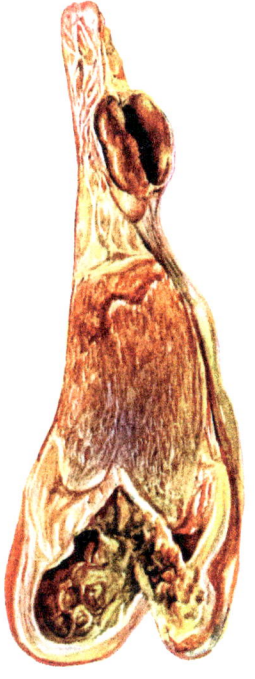

Kr.-G. Nr. 45.

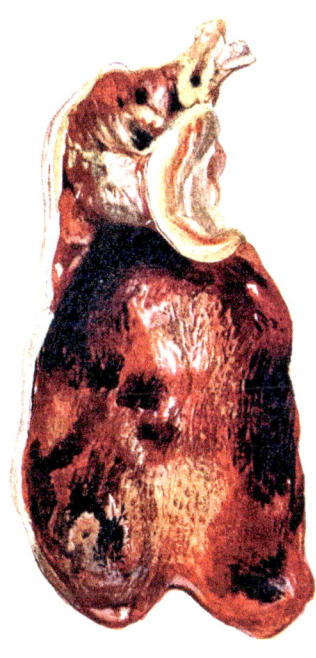

Kr.-G. Nr. 46.

Case 47
Table 39
35-year-old female from Gnadau
Admission: May 29, 1905
Surgery: May 30, 1905
Discharged: June 30, 1906, Cured

For years, agonizing pain under the right costal region. No jaundice.

Surgery: No enlarged liver. Stones in the inflamed gallbladder can be left in and removed following discharge.

Figure 1: Gallbladder, small size, slight edema.

Case 49
Table 39
38-year-old female from Wismar
Admission: May 28, 1905
Surgery: May 29, 1905
Discharge: July 9, 1905

One-year history of abdominal pain. One week of jaundice.

Large distended gallbladder with a stone located in the neck of the gallbladder creating an ulcer.

Duration of Surgery: 30 minutes. (Easy surgery)

Figure 3: Large hydrops of gallbladder. Ulceration at the neck (small stones?).

Case 50
Table 39
50-year-old female (from Russia)
Admission: 6-5-1905
Surgery: 6-5-1905
Discharge: 7-27-1905

Syphilis for 2 years. Right upper quadrant pain. No dark urine. No jaundice.

Surgery: Small shrunken, but thick gallbladder with stones and two ulcer formations at the neck. Difficult ectomy. Seven small ulcers at the neck. Choledochus looks normal. Severe adhesions and bleeding.

OR Time: 1 hour

Histology: Chronic inflammation. Cirrhotic liver.

Figure 4: Thick, small, gallbladder, two ulcers at the neck of gallbladder.

Summarized Case Report

Case 51
Table 39
41-year-old widow of salesman from Chemvitz
Admission: 6-26-1905
Surgery: 6-28-1905
Discharge: 7-12-1905

Colicky pain for years in the right upper quadrant. Had to spend 4 weeks in bed. No fever, but developed icterus and fever lately and vomiting. Poor general condition.

Surgery: Adhesions, no enlarged liver but severe adhesions around the enlarged gallbladder. Removal of gallbladder contained pus and a large stone. Severe bleeding from liver bed. Need multiple drainage.

Duration of Surgery: 30 minutes

Histology: Small gallbladder, small but very thick wall with an ulcer. No tumor cells, free postoperative course.

Two weeks later, sudden death (embolism?).

The information for Case 2 was missing from the Kehr book.

Figure 5: Small, thick-walled gallbladder with several ulcerations, containing stones.

Table 39

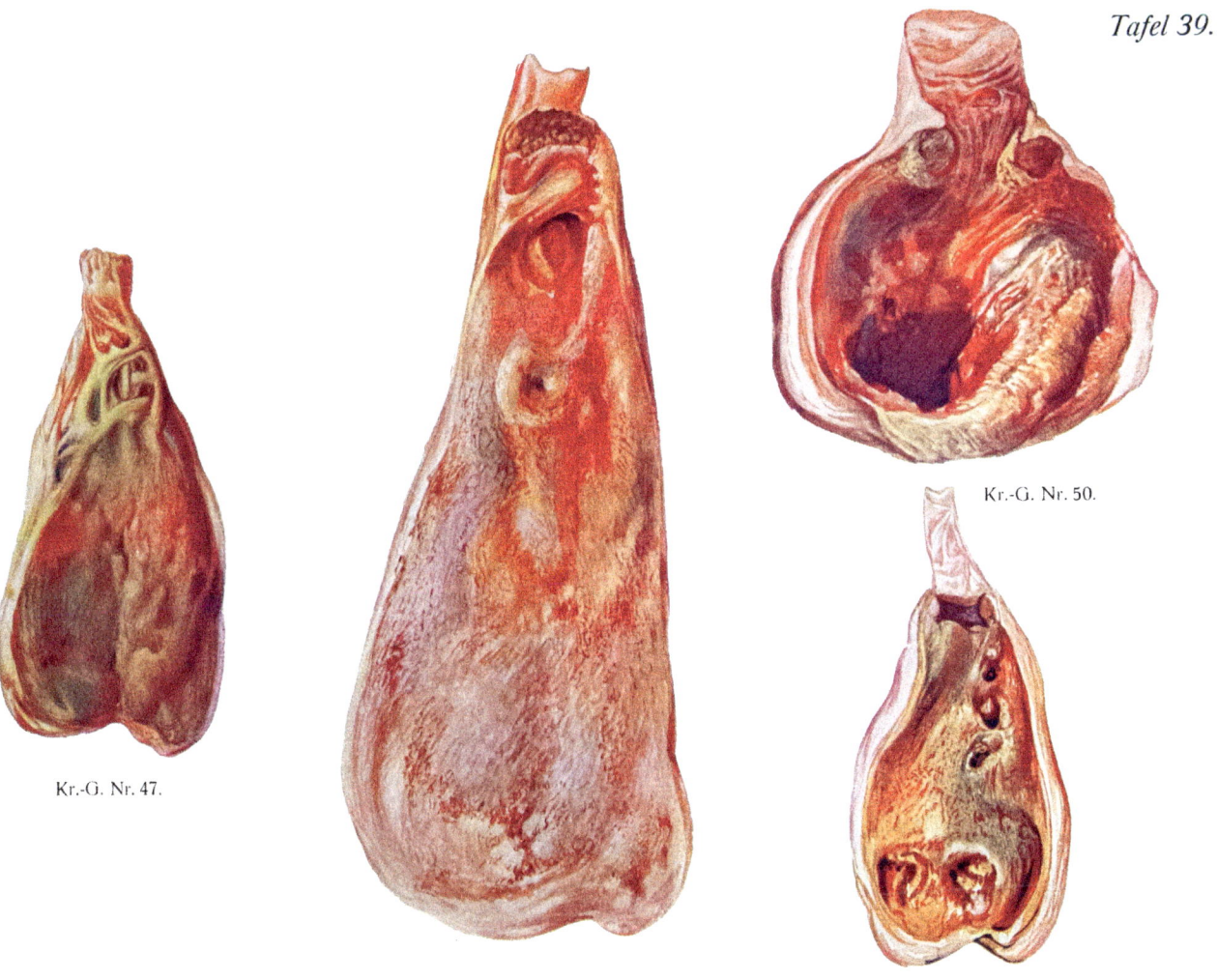

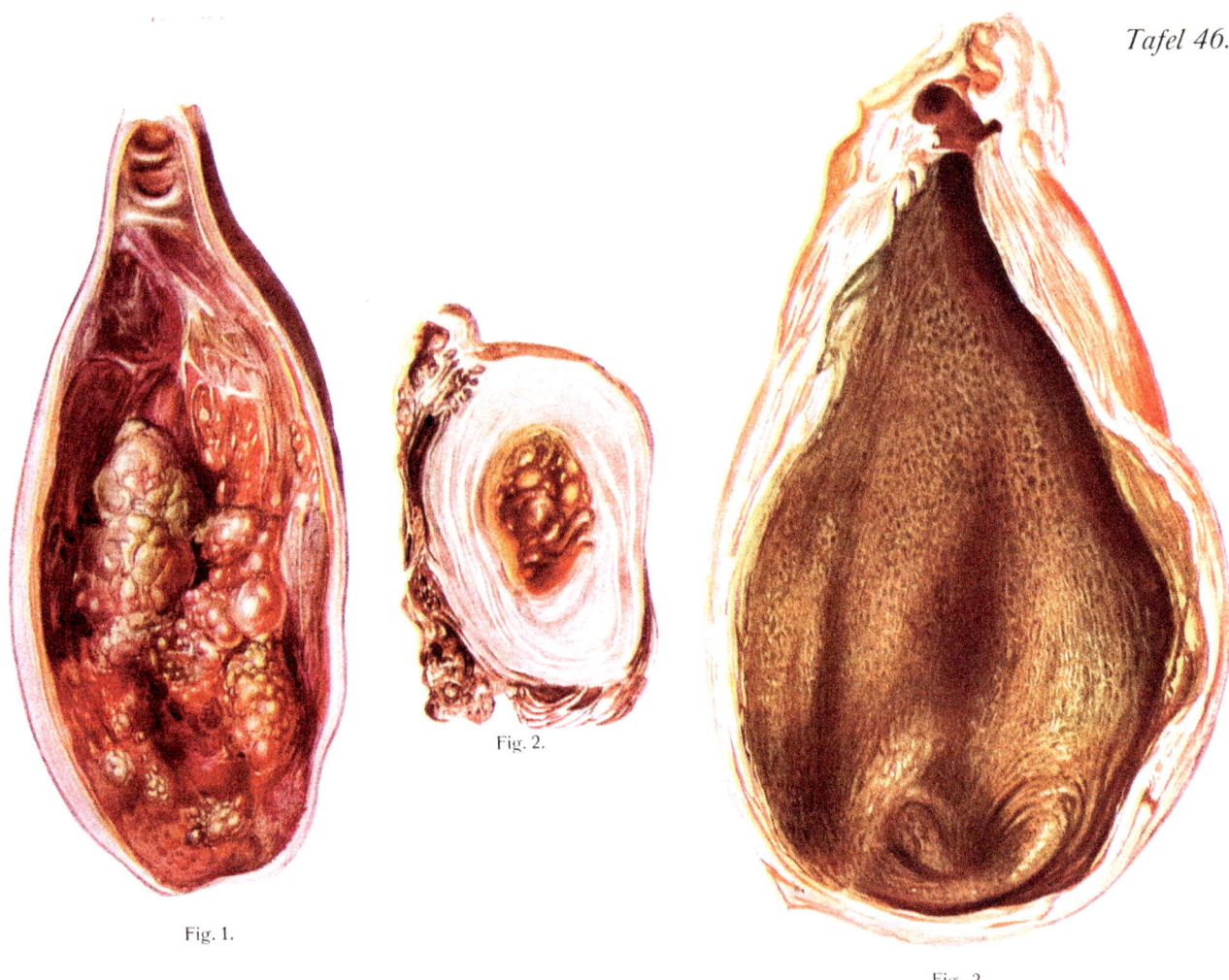

Gallbladders with Carcinomas

Figure 1: A thick gallbladder wall with an ulcer in the neck of the thick-walled gallbladder.

Figure 2: Huge gallbladder with pseudo-membrane appearance. Fibrinous collection on the inside. (In detailed descriptions of these six cases, three were missing.)

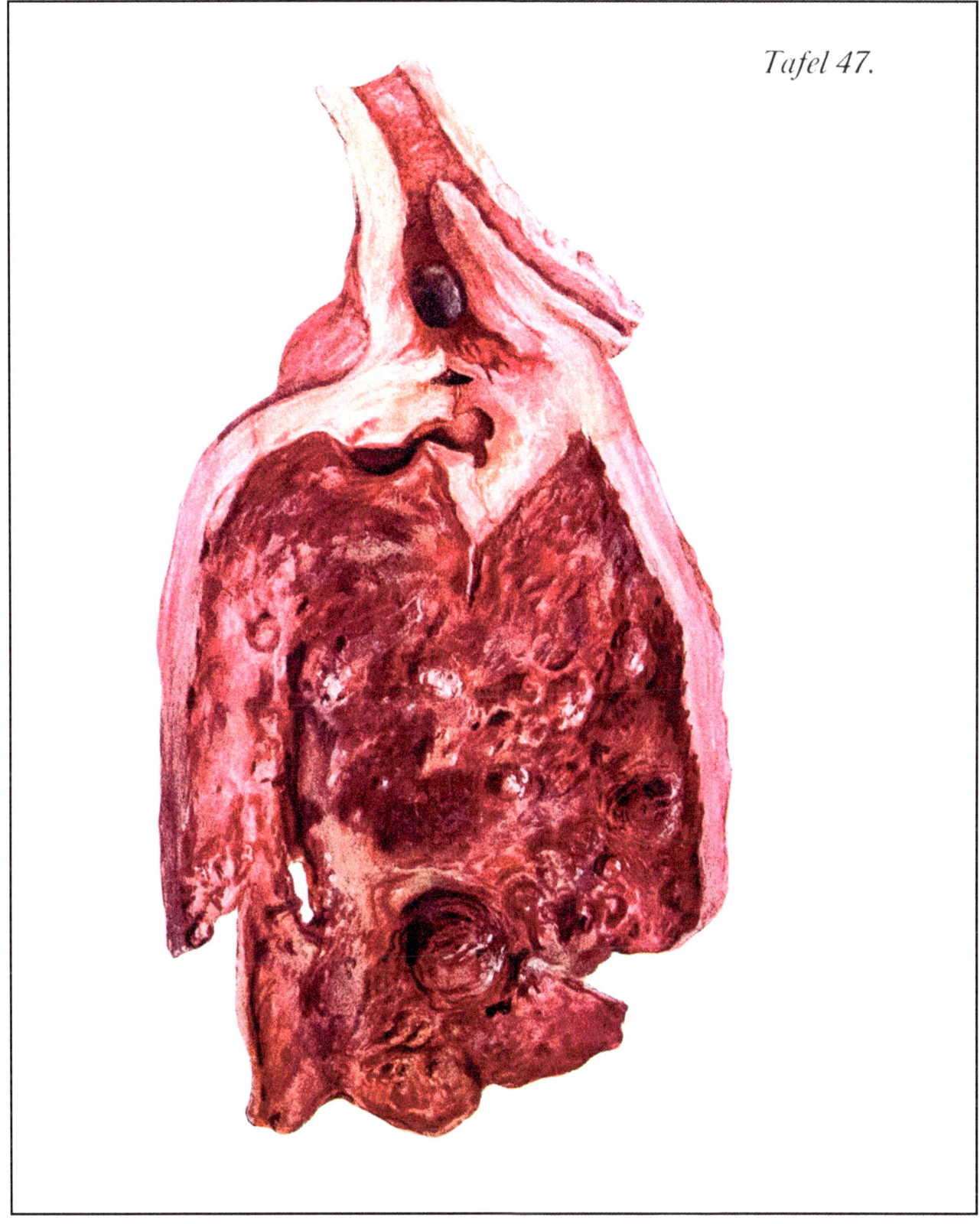

Figure 47: Dilated, hemorrhagic gallbladder with thick wall

Histology: Carcinoma

Unfortunately, our artist had no time to sketch some specimens with a visible cancer because surgeons removed the gallbladder and if it was suspicious for malignancy, it was immediately handed over to the stand-by pathologist. No time was available for drawings – except in a few cases.

(It was difficult to make drawings in suspected or obvious cancerous gallbladder with a standing by pathologist. – Dr. Kehr).

Necrosis of hyperemic thick wall. Carcinoma.

(According to Aschoff, stones rarely cause carcinomas, but rather inflammations. Cited by Kehr.)

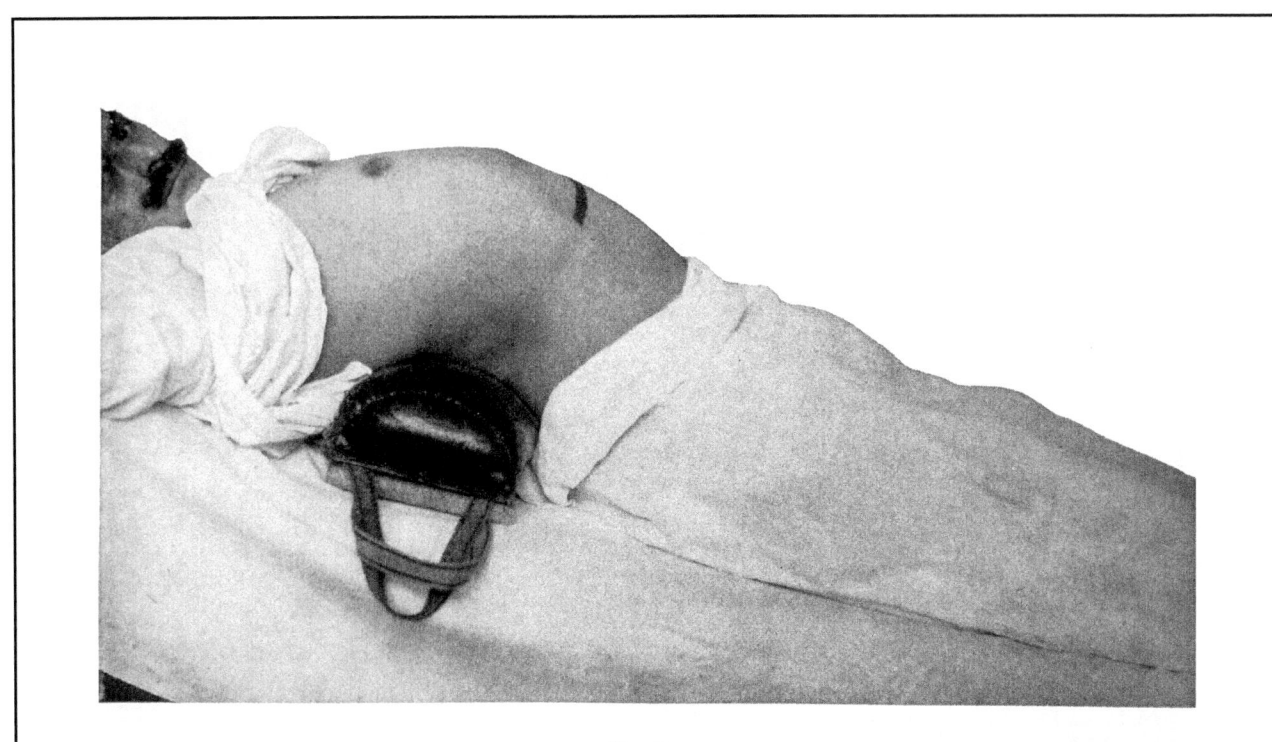

Fig. 2.

Preoperative Position

An insufflatable bag is inserted on the table and distended to increase the rib-cage abdomen angulation.

Surgery 6

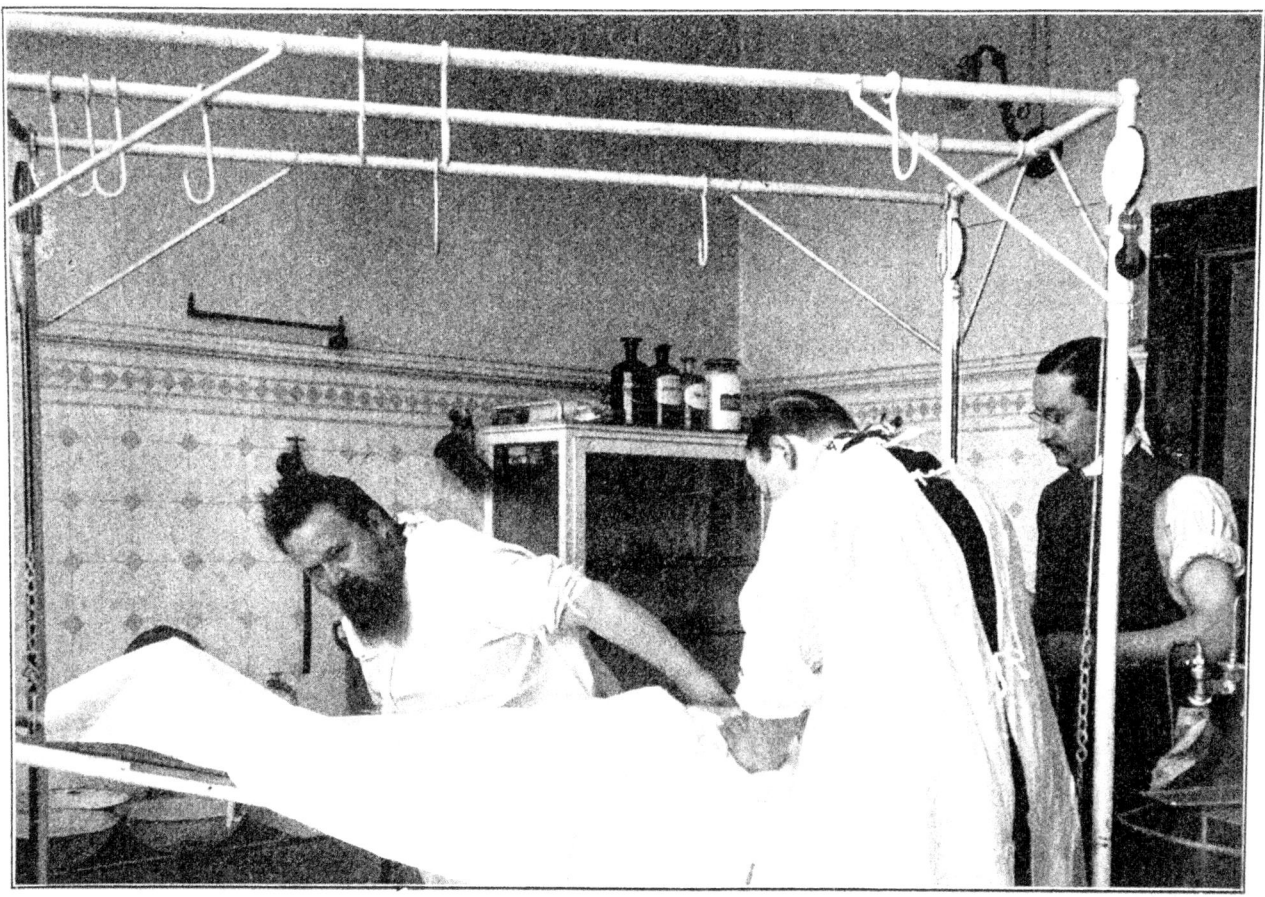

Fig. 99. Stellung des Operateurs beim Abtasten des D. cysticus und choledochus.
(Die linke Hand ist in die Bauchhöhle eingeführt).

Translation:
Dr. Kehr during surgery. Left hand palpates the cystic duct and common bile duct. Assistant retracts the incision. Anesthesiologist stands by.

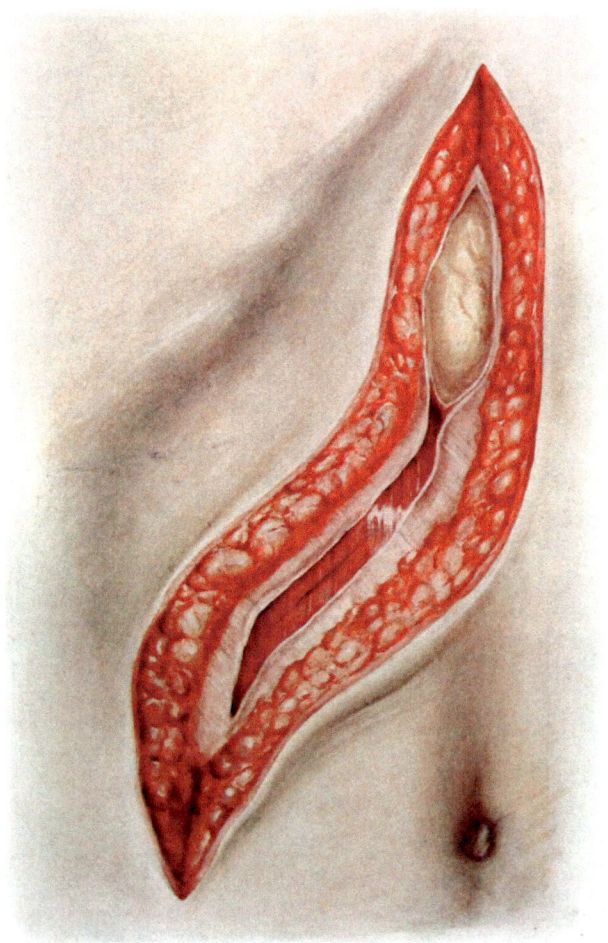
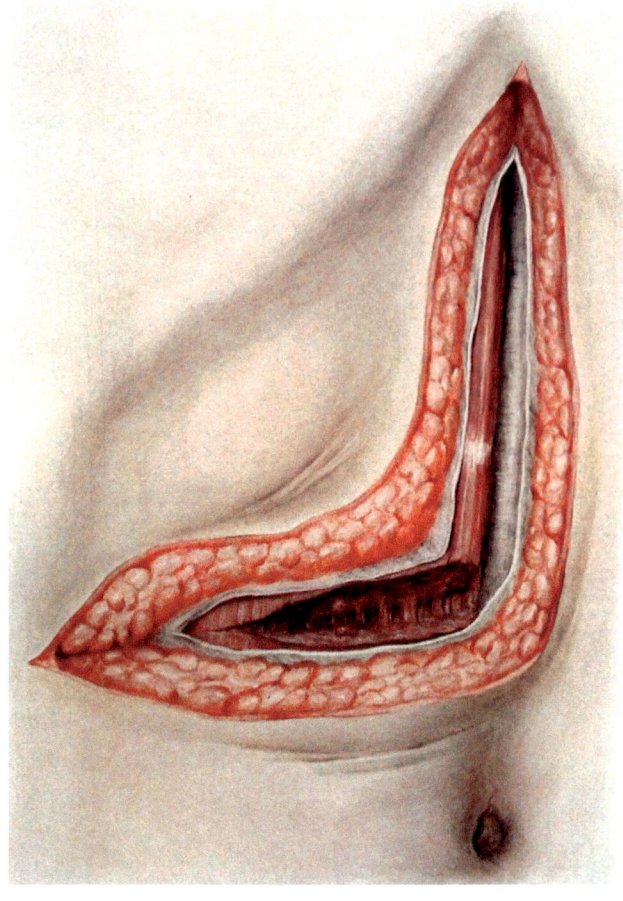

These are the approaches of incisions Kehr recommended

6 Surgery

Tafel 57. **Table 65.**

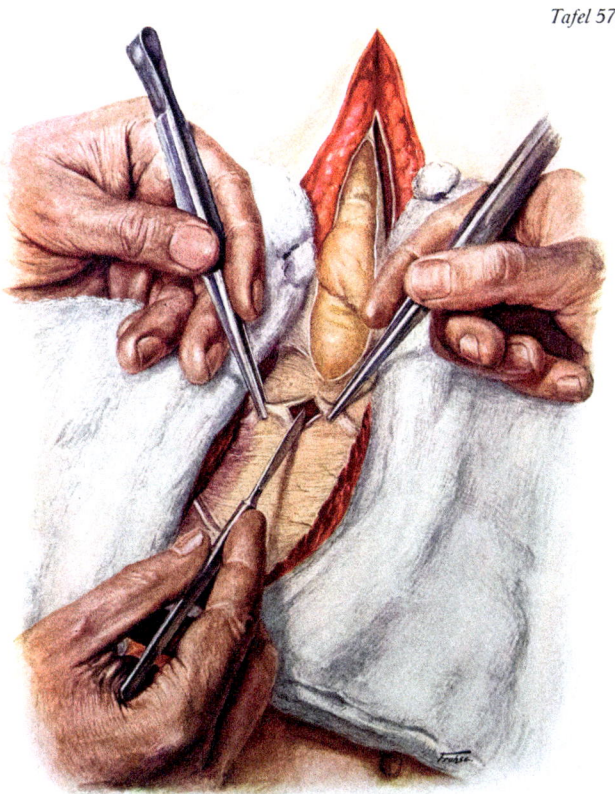

Figure 14. The peritoneum is incised, and the skin and underlying tissues are protected by a wet cloth. The surgeon extends the incision to explore the abdominal cavity.

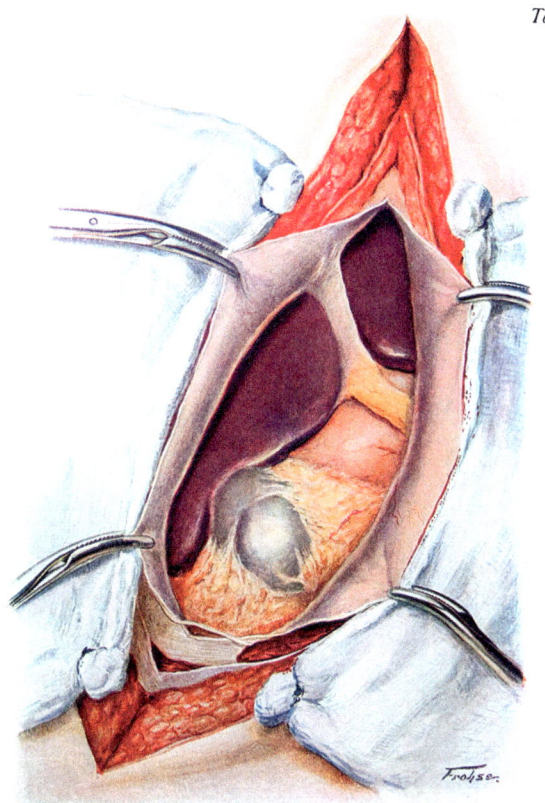

Explored abdominal wall.

Table 66.

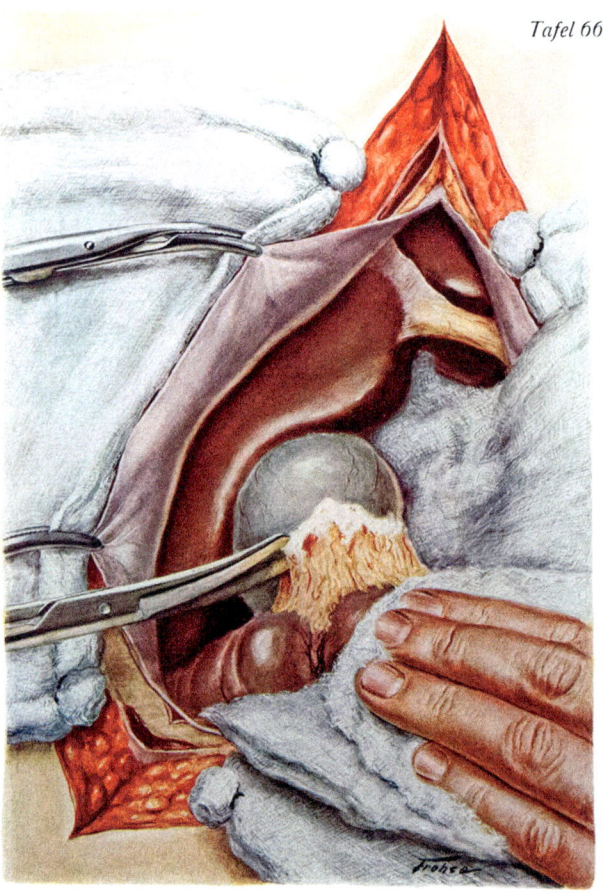

Tafel 66.

Explored patient. The surgeon excises the adhesions from dilated gallbladder with stone. The assistant retracts with left hand. The peritoneum is retracted and clipped to the skin.

Table 68

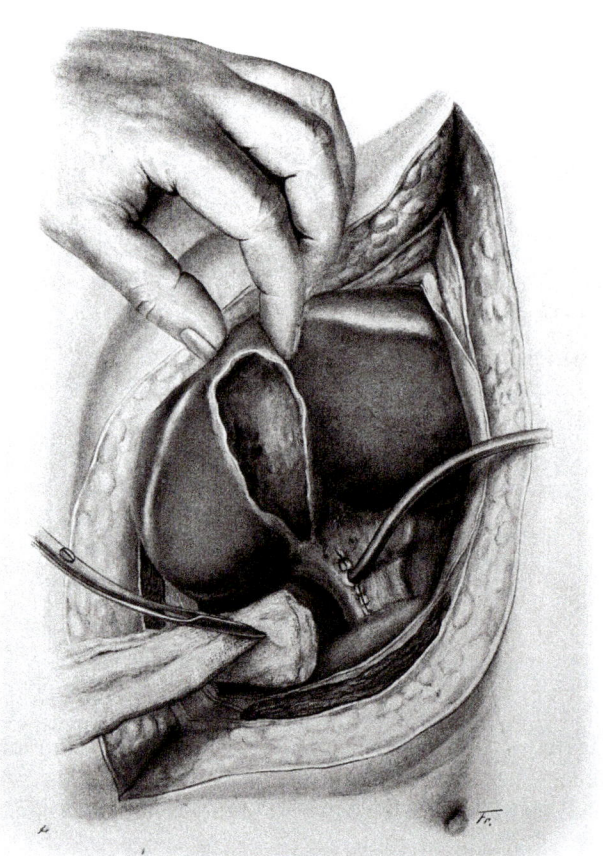

Tafel 68.

Left hand of surgeon is well visible. Black and white drawing during open surgery of surgeon holding posterior wall of the gallbladder. Anterior wall is excised.

Explored dilated choledochus (with stones) sutured over a Kehr T-tube after the calculi were removed.

Summarized Detail of 68 Operated Cases

Female 48 (out of 65)

Age: over 60: 5

Cholecystectomy: 57 (8 cholecystostomy only)

Op Time: Average 50 minutes. 15 cases longer. Max time: 1 hour 15 minutes.

CBD stones: 38

Icterus: 45

Average history: 1–3 years with intermittent icterus and severe colic.

The majority received preop morphine and became addicts.

"Epicrise" summary after case report with long histories and findings, including anomalies and drawings. Referral Dr. mentioned with referral opinions.

65 operated cases described in great detail.

Mortality: 7 Cases (9.3%)

Patient 1. Referred from another surgeon with transected hepatic duct and bile drainage.

Patient 2. 30-year-old with sepsis deep icterus.

Patient 3. 70-year-old cirrhotic liver, fever, and postop pneumonia.

Patient 4. 50-year-old icterus, profuse intraoperative bleeding, postop emboli.

Patient 5. 30-year-old icterus intraoperative severe bleeding, postop emboli.

Patient 6. 44-year-old duodenal injuries with bleeding adhesions, postop cardiac problems.

Patient 7. 54-year-old icterus severe intraoperative bleeding. Death 2 hours postop.

Kehr reported a total number of 2600 biliary cases over 24 years.

Part II
The Gallbladder and Adjacent Structures

History of Endoscopy

Abstract

The first cystoscope through which the image was transmitted by an optical system as well as a distal illumination system was introduced by Nitze. This opened the field in urology and many other areas. Jacobeus took the existing Nitze cystoscope and applied it to intrabdominal examinations in patients with ascites. Thus, the first laparoscopic approach was developed.

Keywords

Endoscopic history · Surgical endoscopy Laparoscopy

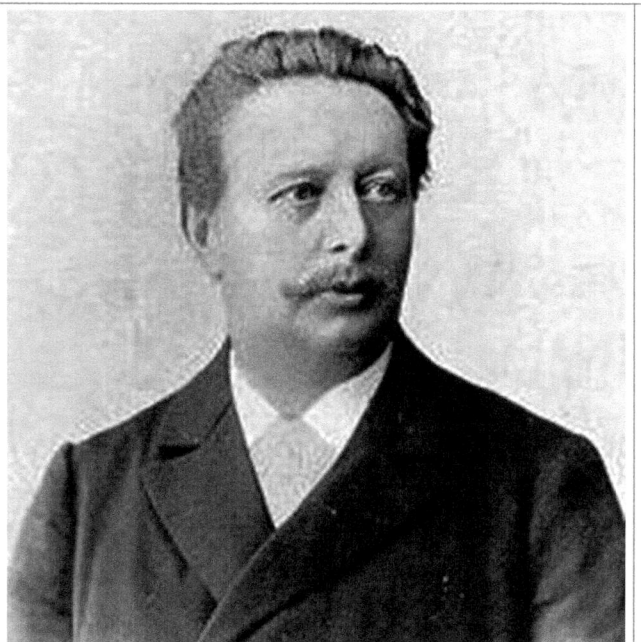 Nitze

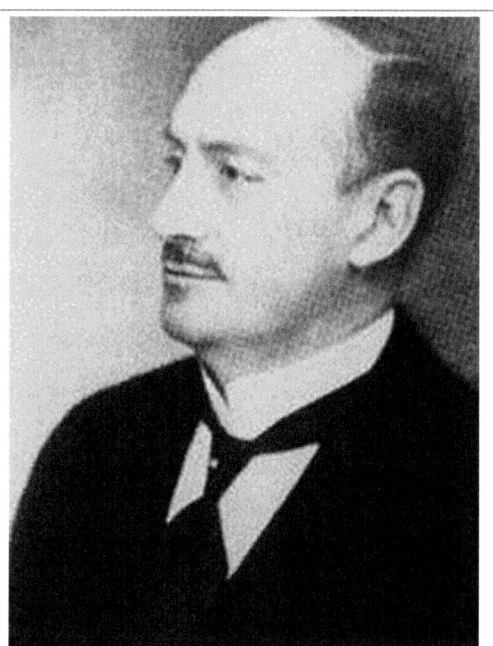 Jacobeus

Maximilian Nitze (1849–1906), Germany

The first cystoscope where the image was transmitted by an optical system as well as a distal illumination system was made by Nitze [1]. One of the largest disease problems in the past for males was the inability to control urination, and therefore the invention of the cystoscopy by Nitze in 1879 opened the field in urology and many other areas. Endoscopic views were also obtained to diagnose or treat abnormalities in the areas of laryngology and proctology.

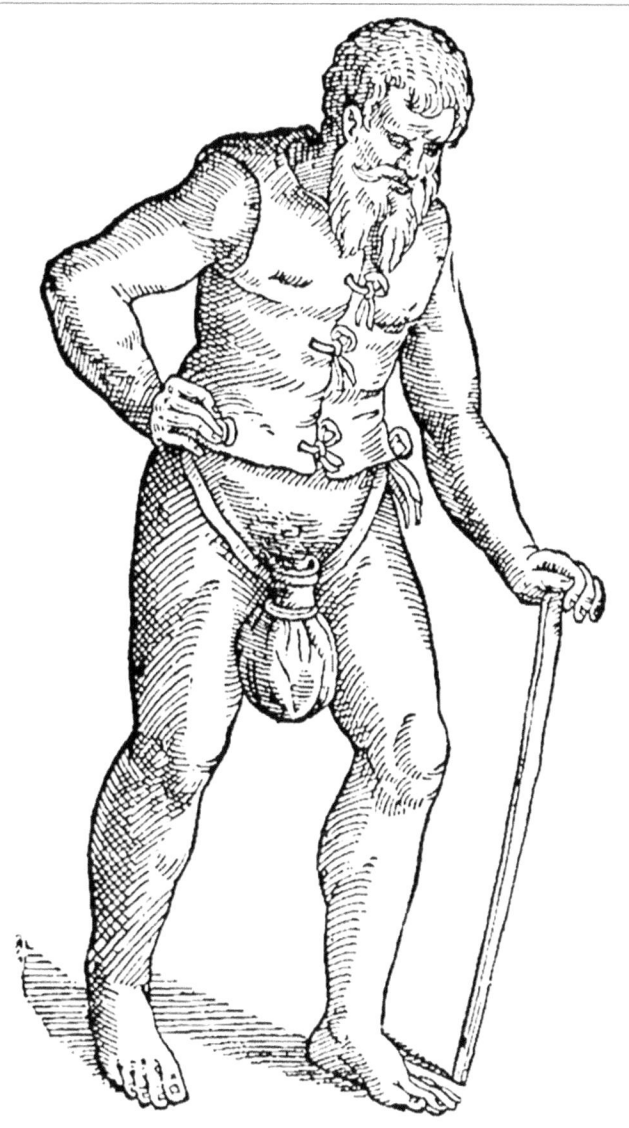

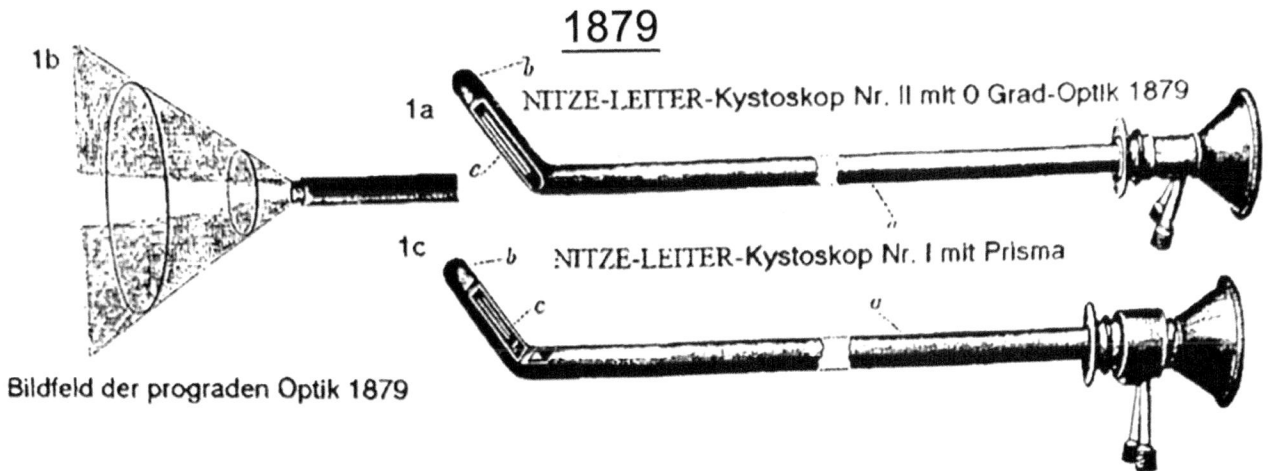

Bildfeld der prograden Optik 1879

Hans Christian Jacobeus [2] (1879–1937), Sweden

He took the existing Nitze cystoscope and, after selecting patients with ascites, the first laparoscopic approach was published. At a later stage, he was able to refine laparoscopy for abdominal diagnostic modalities without ascites using local anesthesia and air insufflation.

References

1. Nitze, M: Eine neue Beobachtung und Untersuchungsmethode d. Harnblase. Wien Med Wochenschr 24:659, 1879.
2. Jacobeus HC: Kurze Ubersicht uber meine Erfahrungen mit der Laparoskopie. Munch Med Wochenschr 58:2017, 1911.

Early Biliary Surgeons

Abstract

On July 15, 1882, Langenbuch successfully removed the gallbladder of a 43-year-old man, thereby performing the first successful cholecystectomy. Ludwig Courvoisier reported in 1890 the successful removal of a CBD stone and created the term choledochotomy. The Swiss surgeon, Theodor Kocher, performed his first cholecystotomy in 1854. In 1881, Halsted performed his first gallbladder operation. A prolonged controversy existed between the advocates of cholecystectomy and those, led by Lawson Tate of London, who supported cholecystotomy.

Keywords

Cholecystectomy · Biliary surgical history
Cholecystotomy

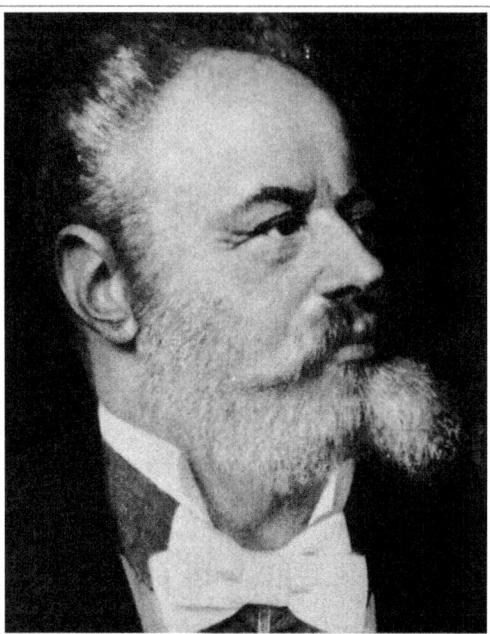

Carl Langenbuch

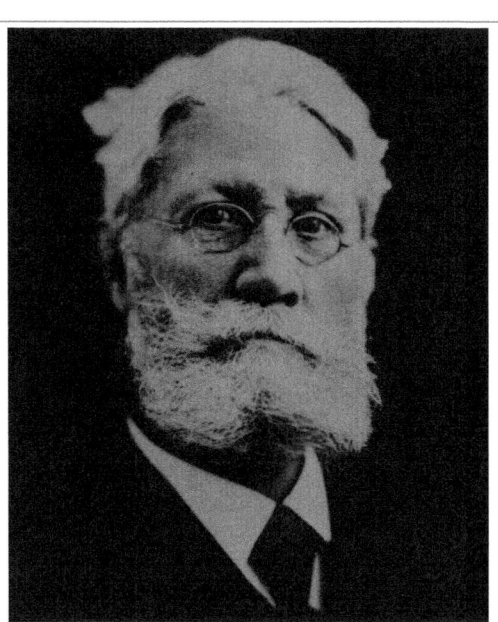

Ludwig Courvoisier

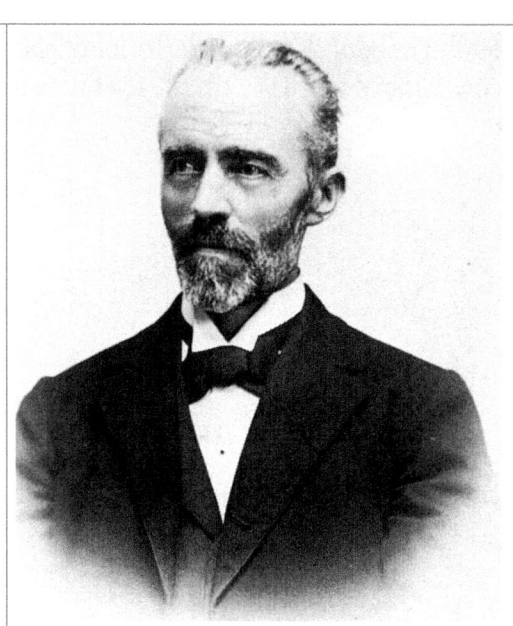

Emil Kocher

While others were pursuing the construction of gallbladder fistulas and direct removal of gallstones, Carl Johann August Langenbuch (1846–1901) of Berlin was preparing himself to completely remove the organ, for he had observed that simple drainage and stone removal gave only temporary relief. Since stones were known to reoccur in the gallbladder, he stated, "they (other surgeons) have busied themselves with the product of the disease, not the disease itself." Langenbuch, who at 27 years of age, had been appointed Director of the Lazarus Hospital Berlin, developed the technique for cholecystectomy through several years of cadaver dissection. On July 15, 1882, he successfully removed the gallbladder of a 43-year-old man who had suffered from biliary colic for 16 years, thereby performing the first successful cholecystectomy and initiating a prolonged controversy between the advocates of cholecystectomy and those, led by Lawson Tate of London, who supported cholecystotomy [1].

In the early years of the twentieth century, operations were hazardous. For example, of 100 cholecystectomies reported in 1897, the mortality was 20%. No specific diagnostic test for biliary tract disease was available and prominent clinical signs such as a tender right upper quadrant with fever and jaundice needed to be present before an operation on the gallbladder could be entertained.

Ludwig Courvoisier (1843–1918) reported in 1890 the successful removal of a CBD stone and created also the terminology of a choledochotomy, as well as the Courvoisier gallbladder (jaundiced, dilated, painless gallbladder with cancer). He also performed the first systematic choledochotomy with an external drain. He worked in Basel, Switzerland, and published the first monograph on the surgery of the biliary system in 1890 and provided also the first detailed description of gallstone ileus [2].

The famous Swiss surgeon, Emil Theodor Kocher (1841–1917), performed his first cholecystotomy in 1854. Using his special approach, the patient survived. It is interesting to note that, in Switzerland, the iodine deficiency at that time was high, creating thyroid disease in large numbers. Kocher received the first Nobel Prize for a surgeon for his outstanding contribution to surgery, particularly in thyroid disease. He also created a new school for biliary surgery with his right subcostal approach [3].

Common duct surgery was still a field for future development. Anesthesia had been in use for only 35 years and Joseph Lister (1827–1912) had visited the United States less than 5 years earlier. Abdominal surgery was truly just being born. In the decade preceding Lister's contributions, 7696 operations were performed at the Massachusetts General Hospital. Two decades later, in 1881, the number had more than tripled to 24,270. In that same year, the year Halsted did his first gallbladder operation, there were 172 operations in more than 5000 admissions to the Charity Hospital in New Orleans. Among these, 72 were amputations, 23 were incisions for abscesses, and 18 were for extraction of bullets; there was only one laparotomy.

References

1. Langenbuch, C. Ein Fall von Exstirpation der Gallenblase wegen chronischer Cholelithiasis. Heilung. Berl Klin Wochenschr 1882; 19: 725–7.
2. Courvoisier, LG, Casuistisch-Statistische Beitrage zur Pathologie und Chirurgie der Gallenwege. Leipzig (Germany); Verlag von FCW Vogel, 1890.
3. Kocher J. Mannskopfgrosses empyrem der gallenblase, Heilung durch incision. Cor-Bl f Schweiz Basel Aerzte 8:577, 1878.

Early American Surgeons

Abstract

Drs. William and Charles Mayo visited Dr. Kehr in Berlin. A variety of tubes were devised for common duct drainage, but the rubber T- tube, introduced by Kehr in the early 1900s proved to be the one universally adopted. In 1886, Justus Ohage of Saint Paul, MN, operated on a 34-year-old woman with a three-month history of right upper quadrant pain, thus performing the first cholecystectomy in the United States. Frank Glenn, MD, published a famous atlas of biliary tract surgery in 1963 with magnificent drawings of the anatomy and the various vascular and ductal anomalies as well as diseases of the biliary tract and palliative operations.

Keywords

Biliary surgical history · Mayo brothers Cholecystectomy

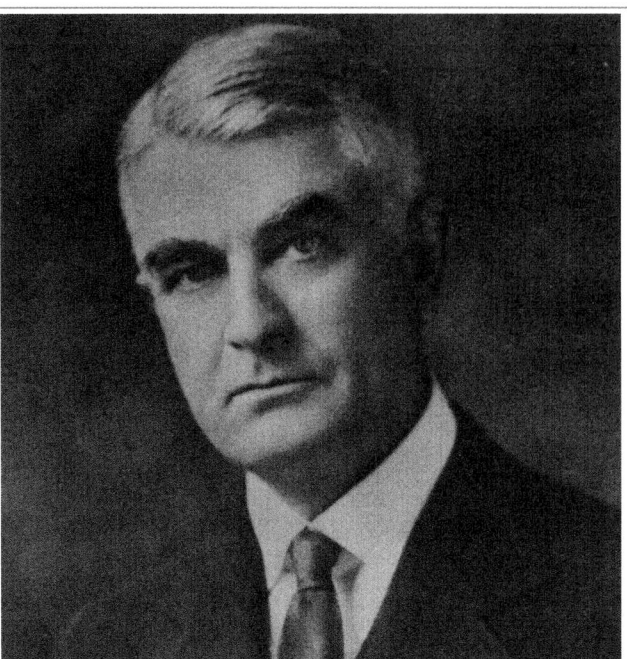
William Mayo

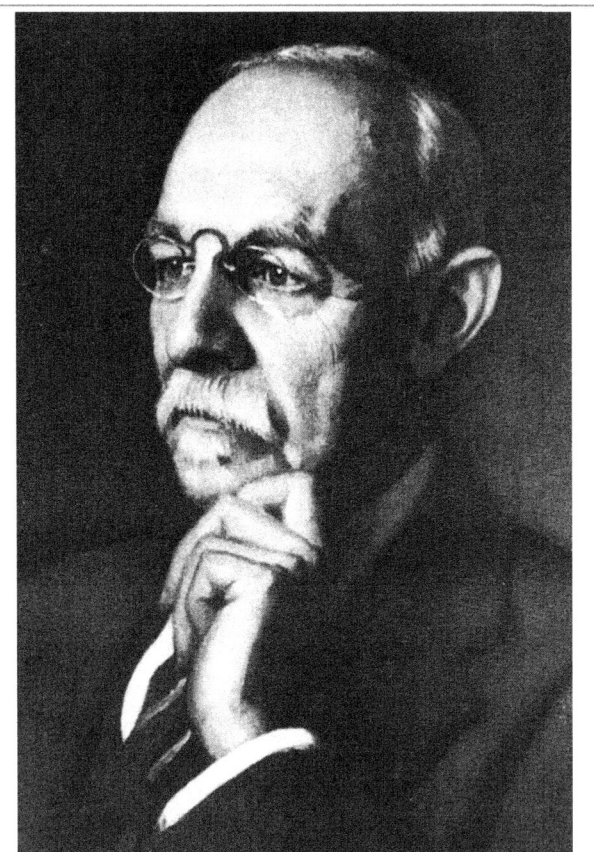
William S. Halsted

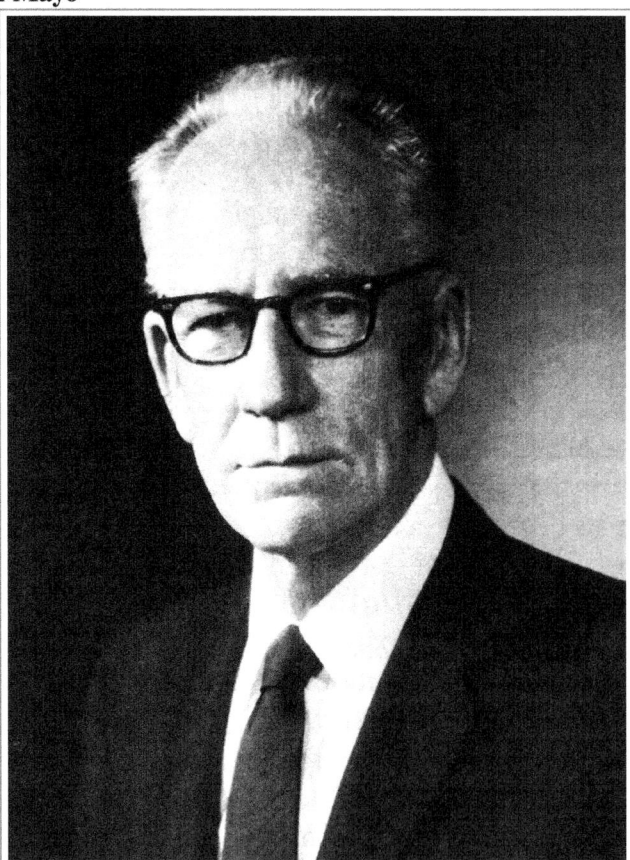
Frank Glenn

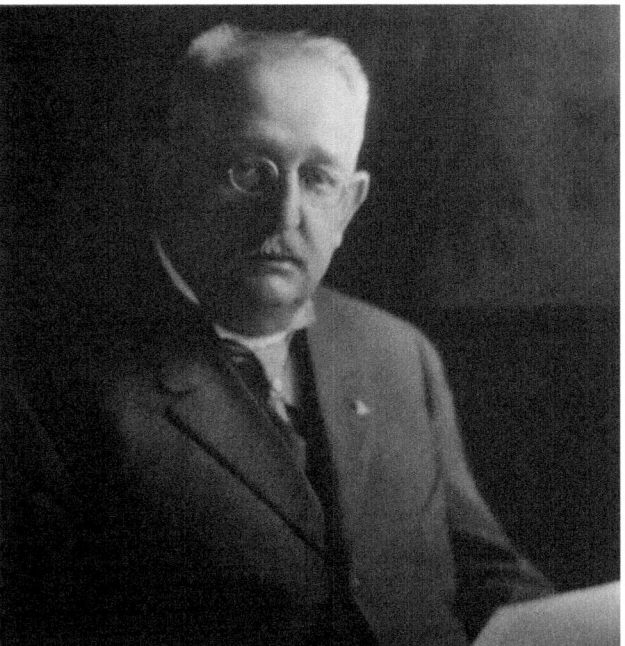

Justus C. Ohage

An important figure in American surgery, William Mayo (1861–1939) was born in Rochester, NY, and attended the University of Michigan School of Medicine. He moved to New York and obtained his postgraduate education, taking several annual leaves to visit centers in the United States and overseas. He practiced with his father, William, and his brother, Carl Mayo (1865–1939). Together, they established the Mayo Clinic, one of the most important centers in medical training and research. He was a leading personality in various associations, including the American Medical Association, the Society of Clinical Surgery, and the American College of Surgeons. He was very interested in gastric surgery as well as rectal disorders, particularly cancer. He published the first cholecystectomy in 1893. With his brother, Carl, he visited Dr. Kehr in Berlin. During his activities, over 2100 papers were published [1].

In 1881, William S. Halsted (1852–1922) performed his first biliary operation in Albany, New York, on his elderly mother, who was desperately ill with jaundice, fever, and an abdominal mass. He surgically incised the mass, releasing pus and gallstones from the gallbladder. She recovered from this acute illness only to succumb years later to symptoms related to a ball-valve stone in the common duct [2].

One of the early problems of biliary surgery pertained to methods of closing or draining the common duct after exploration. Halsted advocated that a bile-tight closure of the duct made it unnecessary to routinely drain the common bile duct after exploration, a practice also advocated by a number of Halsted's trainees. Halsted also experimented with drainage of the common duct via the cystic duct, a technique that found few followers. A variety of tubes were devised for common duct drainage, but the rubber T-tube, introduced by Kehr in the early 1900s proved to be the one universally adopted.

The first major contribution was an answer to Halsted's admonition that "some sure and simpler method must be devised for determining positively the presence of stones of the ductus choledochus after excision of the gallbladder." In Argentina in 1931, Mirizzi developed the concept of operative cholangiography by introducing iodized oil (Lipiodol) into the duct at operation and recommended the procedure as giving "precise results concerning the causes of biliary obstruction and the indications for common duct exploration." The technique was quickly taken up in this country by those who advocated the routine use of operative cholangiography with cholecystectomy, a proposal still being debated today!

Justus Christoph Ohage (1849–1935), born in Hanover, Germany, in 1849, escaped from home with two of his buddies and ended up in the United States. He was accepted into the volunteer infantry and became a soldier in the US Army. He began his studies at the University of Missouri, and then settled in St. Paul, Minnesota. As a physician, he contacted William Mayo and knew about Langenbuch, who performed the first cholecystectomy 4 years earlier. There were so many patients with gallstone disease. He experimented with cholecystectomies in animals. In 1886, he operated on a 34-year-old woman with a 3-month history of right upper quadrant pain. The surgery was done under ether narcosis and he was able to remove a large, thin gallbladder with 135 stones. The patient was discharged on the 13th postoperative day and lived until age 80. Ohage eventually left surgery and became active in medical society [3].

Frank Glenn (1901–1982) published a famous atlas of biliary tract surgery in 1963 with magnificent drawings of the anatomy and the various anomalies as well as diseases of the biliary tract and palliative operations. The total number of Glenn's biliary surgical cases was in the vicinity of 10,000, the largest experience in the country [4].

References

1. Mayo, WJ, Surgery of the Gall-bladder, cystic and common ducts with report of seven cases operated upon. JAMA 1893; 21:301–2.
2. Halsted, Contributions to the Surgery of the Bile Passages especially of the Common Bile Duct, Boston Med and Surg J, 1891, 141: 645–654.
3. Ohage, JC, The surgical treatment of diseases of the gall-bladder. Medical News 1887; 50:233–6.
4. Glenn, F, Grafe WR Jr. Historical events in biliary tract surgery. Arch Surg 1966; 93:848–52.

Endoscopy

Abstract

The persistent pioneering efforts of Rudolph Schindler with the semi-rigid gastroscope opened a new era of gastric pathology. The cannulation of the ampulla of Vater by McCune et al. in 1968 and Oi in 1970 added another technique for detailed radiologic examination of the biliary system (ERCP). The idea of a choledochoscope was suggested by Bakes, and such an instrument was developed by Melver of New York in 1941. These diagnostic procedures have been of great assistance in the diagnosis of biliary tract disease and have helped to reduce, but sadly not to eliminate one of the most unfortunate events in biliary surgery—the retained common duct stone.

Keywords

Endoscopic history · ERCP · Choledochoscope Stone extraction

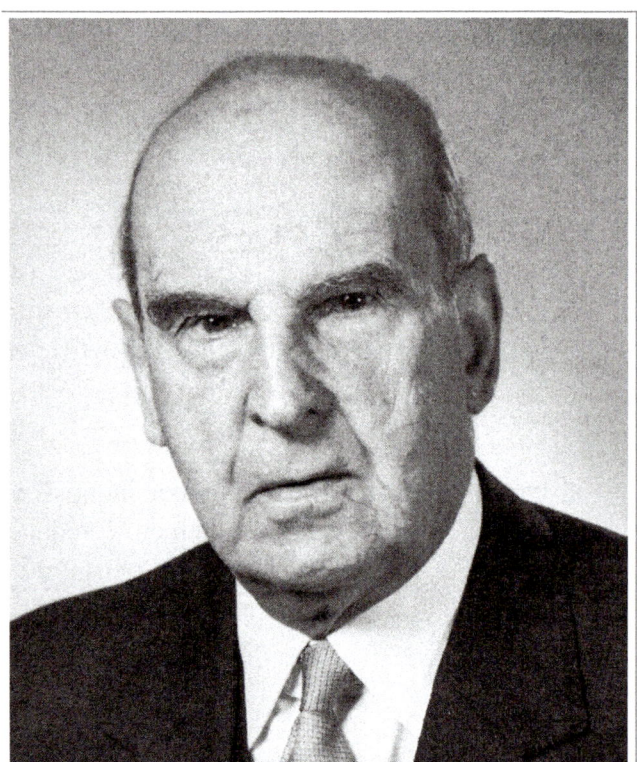
Hans Wildegans

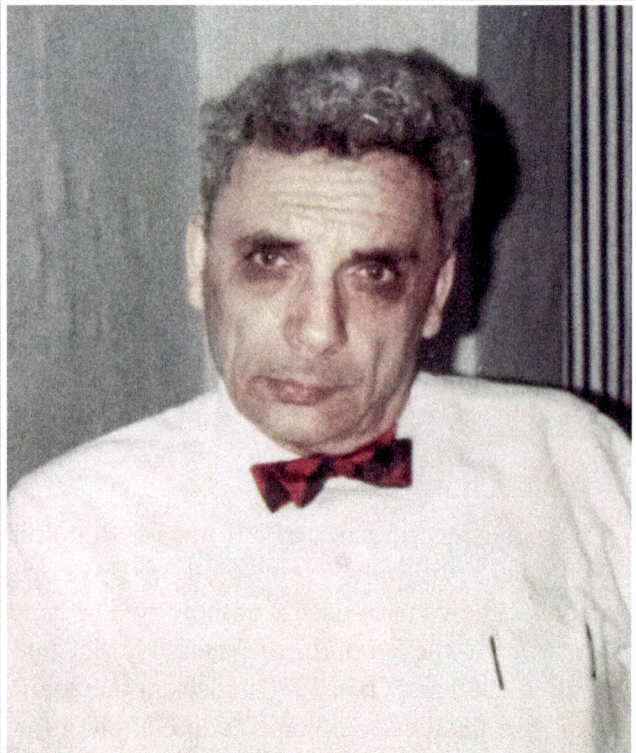
Clarence Schein

The persistent pioneering efforts of Rudolph Schindler (1888–1968) with the semi-rigid gastroscope opened a new era of gastric pathology [1]. The present era of flexible endoscopy began with a publication by Curtiss et al. in 1956 and the introduction of the fiber-optic gastroscope by Hirschowitz et al. in 1957. The development of the Olympus fiber-optic duodenoscope 1968 was a remarkable advance. The cannulation of the ampulla of Vater by McCune et al. in 1968 and Oi in 1970 added another technique for detailed radiologic examination of the biliary system (ERCP) [2]. These diagnostic procedures have been of great assistance in the diagnosis of biliary tract disease and have helped to reduce, but sadly not to eliminate, one of the most unfortunate events in biliary surgery—the retained common duct stone.

Finding one or more stones remaining in the common bile duct after what had been considered a careful and complete biliary exploration has encouraged surgeons to turn to other than reoperation to make stones disappear. The severe irritation and pain caused by volatile solutions such as ether or chloroform limited their use, but the principle was reintroduced in 1972 by J. Way et al., who proposed a solution of cholic acid [3], and by Gardener who suggested a solution of heparin [4]. Later the compound monooctanoin was found to be more effective and less toxic. Unfortunately, the percentage of retained stones that could be dissolved by such treatments remained small.

In the 1960s, Mazzariello, another Argentine surgeon, reported the successful extraction of stones through the mature T-tube sinus tract using specially designed stone forceps [5]. Burhenne reported over 600 cases of duct stones successfully extracted under fluoroscopic control [6].

The idea of a choledochoscope was suggested by Bakes, and such an instrument was developed by Melver of New York in 1941 [7].

Hans Wildegans (1888–1967), of Berlin, further developed the rigid choledochoscope in 1953 and reported an extensive experience in 1960 [8]. George Berci, in 1960, adapted the Hopkins lens system to the rigid scope and greatly improved the visual image and the effectiveness of the instrument [9]. Video-choledochoscopy by either the rigid or flexible choledochoscope is another technique that can assist in minimizing the incidence of retained common duct stones particularly in cases of multiple stones. Successful extraction of stones using flexible choledochoscopy introduced through the T-tube sinus tract has also been reported, but not widely used.

Biliary tract disease, so commonly encountered, is so readily responsive to the local manual manipulations of the surgeon. This provided a field of surgery that developed quickly after general anesthesia lessened pain and Listerism reduced infection to a tolerable level. Writing in the early 1980s, William Longmire (1914–2003) envisioned that "the surgeon must be prepared, probably in the not-too-distant future, to abandon the most commonly performed intra-abdominal operation and move on to other fields of biliary tract lithiasis that respond to the innovations of dietary and/or medical management" [10].

In the early 1980s the revolution spawned by the laparoscopic approach to gallbladder disease had not been appreciated but was on the horizon [2]. Beginning in 1970, Clarence Schein and George Berci collaborated and corresponded for the next 50 years concerning biliary surgery and especially intraoperative cholangiography and choledochoscopy [11]. Biliary surgery was Schein's major interest. He established a unique teaching system for surgical residents at Montefiore Hospital in New York, NY. He published his famous book on acute cholecystitis [12] in 1972 with 629 references. Over 200 publications by Clarence Schein were accepted by periodic journals. Dr. Schein was interested in reading surgical authors in their original language, and therefore he started to learn German to be able to read the classical authors in their original tongue. His other major contribution was to music; he played the clarinet.

References

1. Berci G, Forde KA. History of endoscopy: What lessons have we learned from the past? *Surg Endosc.* 2000;14(1):5-15. https://doi.org/10.1007/s004649900002
2. Ibid.
3. Way LW. The national cooperative gallstone study and chenodiol. Gastroenterology 1983;84:648-51.
4. Glenn F, Grafe WR. Historical Events in Biliary Tract Surgery. *Arch Surg.* 1966;93(5):848-852. https://doi.org/10.1001/archsurg.1966.01330050152025
5. Burhenne HJ. The technique of biliary stone extraction. Radiology 1974; 113: 567-72.
6. Ibid.
7. Glenn F, Grafe WR. Historical Events in Biliary Tract Surgery. *Arch Surg.* 1966;93(5):848-852. https://doi.org/10.1001/archsurg.1966.01330050152025
8. Wildegans, H., Grenzen der cholangiographie und aussichten der endoskopie der tiefen gallenwege. Med Klinik,: 48:1270-1272, 1953.
9. Berci, G., Intraoperative and Postoperative Biliary Endoscopy (Choledochoscopy), Endoscopy 21:299-384, 1989.
10. Longmire, WP Historic Landmarks in Biliary Surgery. *South Med J.* 1982;75(12):1548-1550.
11. Schein, CJ, Biliary Endoscopy, Surg 65:1004, 1969.
12. Ibid.

Laparoscopy

Abstract

The contributions of Heinz Kalk in Germany and John Ruddock in the United States were seminal in the development of laparoscopic approaches to the biliary tract.

Keywords

Laparoscopy · Endoscopy · Endoscopic history

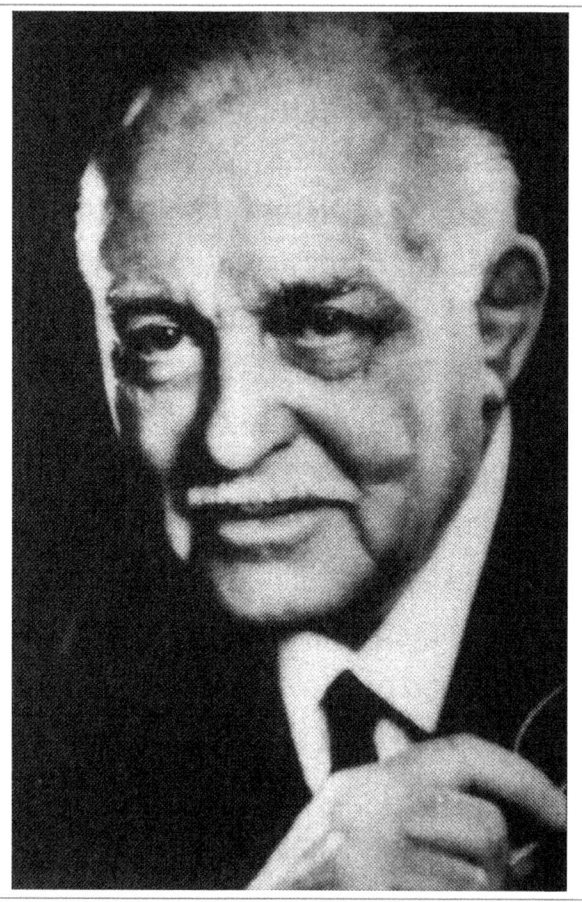
Heinz Kalk

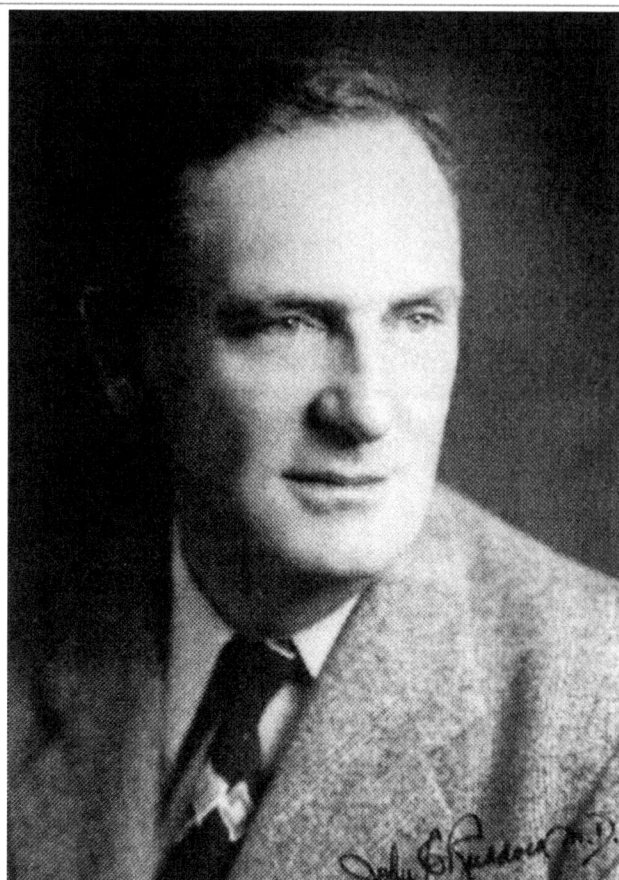
John Ruddock

Heinz Kalk (1895–1973), Germany

Kalk [1] refined the laparoscopic system and, using local anesthesia, performed and published several thousand successful cases. Major indications were liver and pancreatic disease and intra-abdominal carcinomas, as well as biopsies under visual control with coagulation of bleeders. He introduced the various degrees of laparoscopes. He published 2000 successful cases in 1951.

John Ruddock (1891–1964), USA

Ruddock [2] served with the US Army and was a Commander in the US Navy during World War II. After retirement as an internist, he became interested in laparoscopy. He modified the telescope and the biopsy forceps. He published 2500 successful cases performed under local anesthesia with a standby anesthesiologist.

References

1. Kalk H, Bruhl, W: Leitfaden der laparoskopie und Gastroskopie. Stuttgart, Thieme, 1951.
2. Ruddock, JC: Peritoneoscopy: a critical clinical review. Surg Clin North Am 37:1249, 1957

Advances in Visualization for Laparoscopic Surgery

Abstract

The British physicist, Harold Hopkins, developed a rod lens system in 1959 which was smaller in diameter and produced a brighter image with much more resolution. The work of Hopkins, Berci, and Storz created an entire series of smaller rigid endoscopes with vastly improved performance and made a significant impact on present and future clinical results. The new optical systems connected to a video display generated new areas where previous surgical operations were replaced with endoscopic approaches. The recording of procedures on tape or single images was an additional help in the documentation of cases.

Keywords

Endoscopic light sources · Endoscopic images Video endoscopy

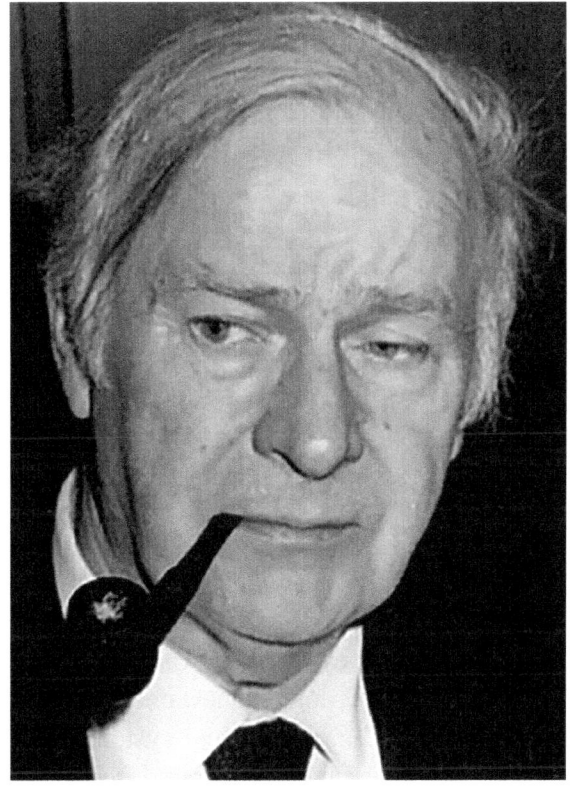

Harold Hopkins

British physicist, Harold Hopkins (1918–1994) developed a rod lens system in 1959 which was smaller in diameter and produced a brighter image with much more resolution. It opened immediately a large number of applications, particularly laparoscopy [1].

The fiber bundle light conduction and the brighter and smaller xenon light source provided safer and better images.

Hopkins also initiated the introduction of the flexible optical and light guiding cables.

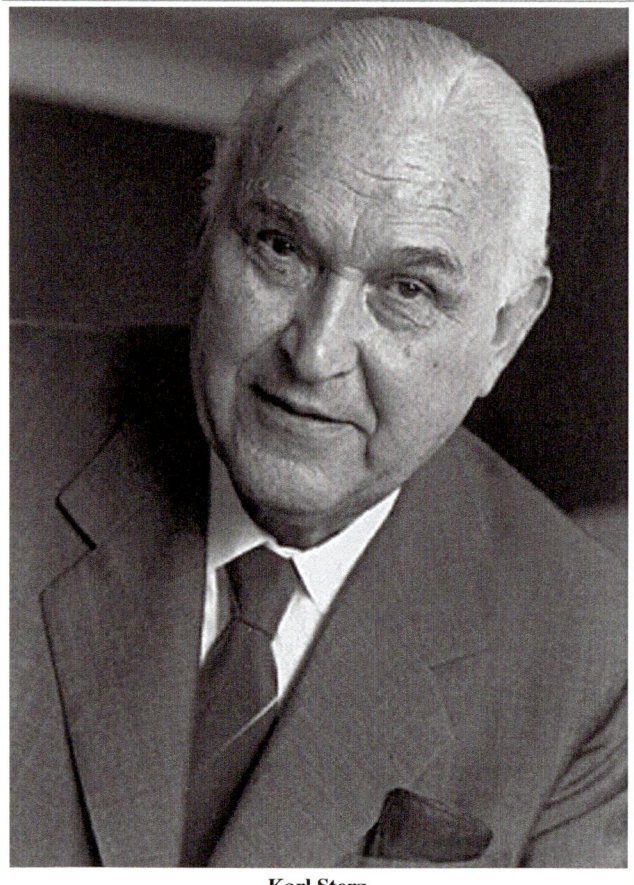
Karl Storz

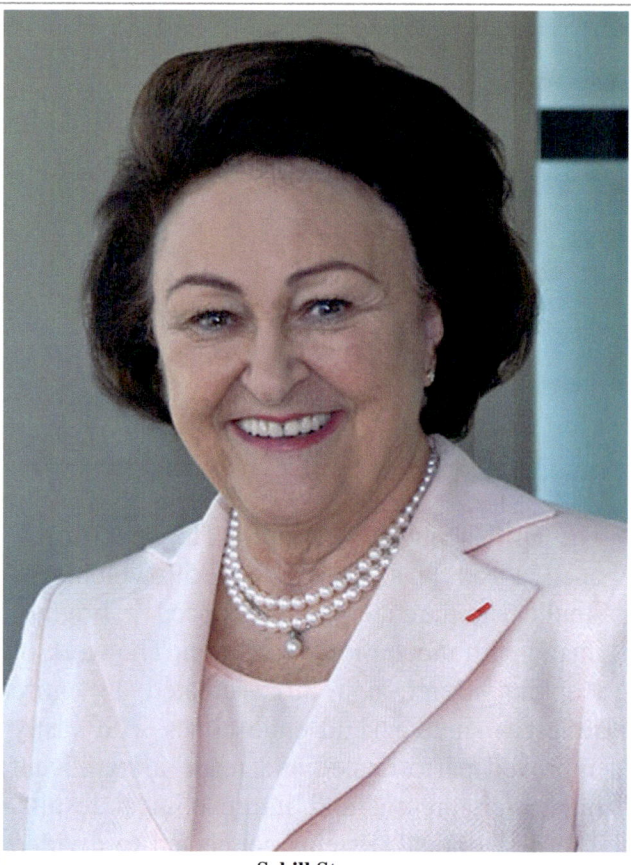
Sybill Storz

Karl Storz (1911–1996) and his daughter, Dr. Sybill Storz, were owners of a small German engineering company. It was recommended by George Berci that they contact Professor Hopkins, thus initiating production of a new endoscopic system (Fig. 12.1). The new optical system covered the entire series of smaller rigid endoscopes with vastly improved performance and made a significant impact on present and future clinical results. It also included the new miniature xenon light source which produced a safer and brighter light as well as a new smaller video system.

Upon receiving prototype samples, a series of new endoscopic tools were designed and/or created. These included pediatric bronchoscopes, esophagoscopes, cystoscopes, and a laparoscope.

The new adult series broncho, cysto-, resecto-, laparo-, thoracoscopes, etc. were made in the early 1960s. A very important area in the early stages was urology with the new operating cysto-resecto-

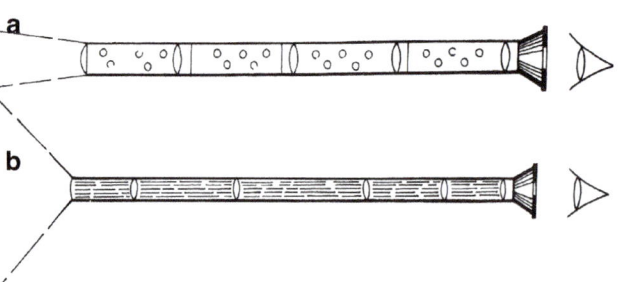

Fig. 12.1 Schematic diagram of telescope. (**a**) Standard lens system. Small optical elements are placed at intervals along the cylinder. (**b**) The Hopkins rod lenses. Glass rods replace the previous air intervals

scope [2, 3]. The new optical systems connected to a video display generated new areas where previous surgical operations were replaced with endoscopic ones reducing hospitalization time and postoperative or recovery days. The design of a new video-intubation system also helped anesthesiology significantly [4].

Looking through an existing monocular telescope eyepiece only, a small image was observed by the examiner (Fig. 12.2). The development of a small TV camera (Fig. 12.3) made it possible to observe the magnified image with both eyes from a secure distance and became an important help in teaching or assistance as well as improving collaboration with the entire operative team. The recording of procedures on tape or single images was an additional help in the documentation of cases.

The abovementioned improvements or replacements played a significant role in the evolution of the next generation of operative video endoscopy.

The enlarged binocular view improved vision and recognition of smaller target areas. The assistant was able to see simultaneously the same area. This became an important teaching tool. The scrub nurse was able to follow the procedure and simultaneous records (simple image, video) could be made (Fig. 12.4).

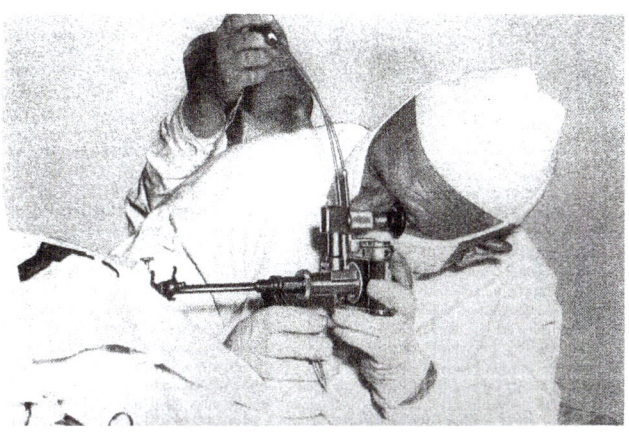

Fig. 12.2 Monocular view of a small image

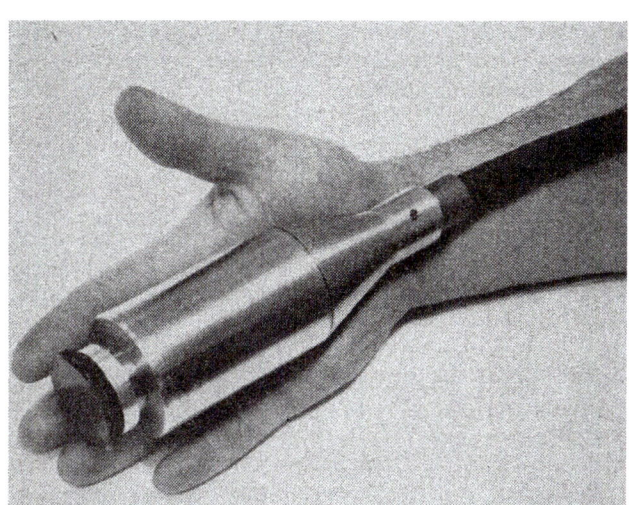

Fig. 12.3 Miniature television camera

Fig. 12.4 Significant magnification of surgical anatomy allowed by modern imaging

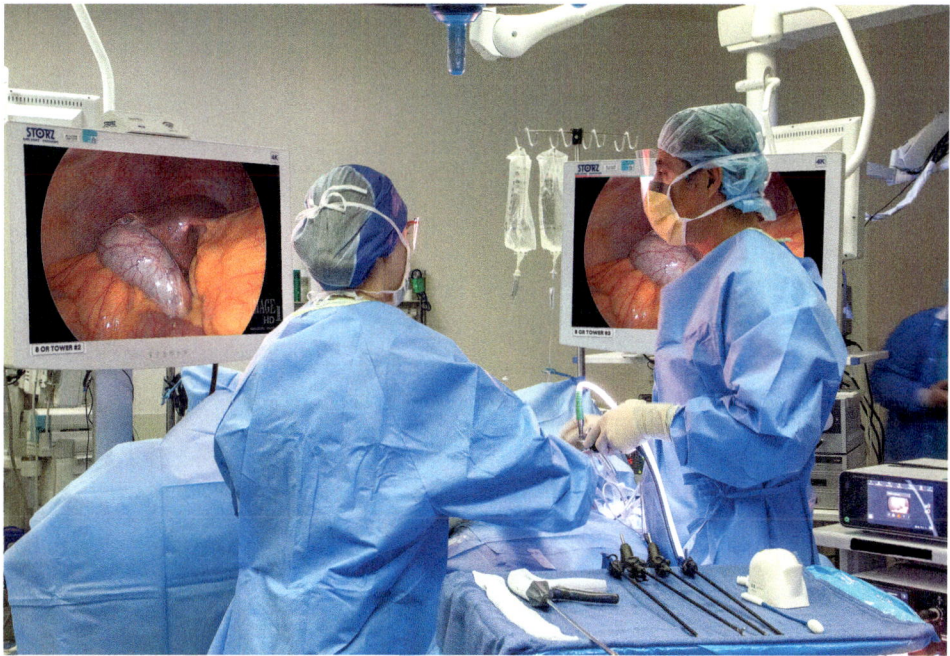

References

1. Hopkins, H., Optical Principles of the Endoscope, G. Berci, Endoscopy, Appleton, Century Crofts, New York, NY, 1976.
2. Berci, G., Davids, J. Endoscopy and Television, Brit Med J 1962, page 1610.
3. Berci, G, Kont, L: A new optical system in endoscopy with special references to cystoscopy. Br J. Urol, 41:564, 1969.
4. A New Video Laryngoscope – An Aid in Intubation and Teaching, Berci, G., Kaplan, M. and Ward, D., J Clin Anesth, 620–626, 2002

Laparoscopic Cholecystectomies

Abstract

There were a number of pioneers in laparoscopic cholecystectomy both in Europe and the United States. These pathfinders developed techniques and played a major role in the teaching of minimal access approaches to gallbladder surgery and the management of common bile duct stones.

Keywords

History of laparoscopic cholecystectomy
Laparoscopic techniques

The original version of this chapter was revised. The correction to this chapter can be found at https://doi.org/10.1007/978-3-030-76845-4_20

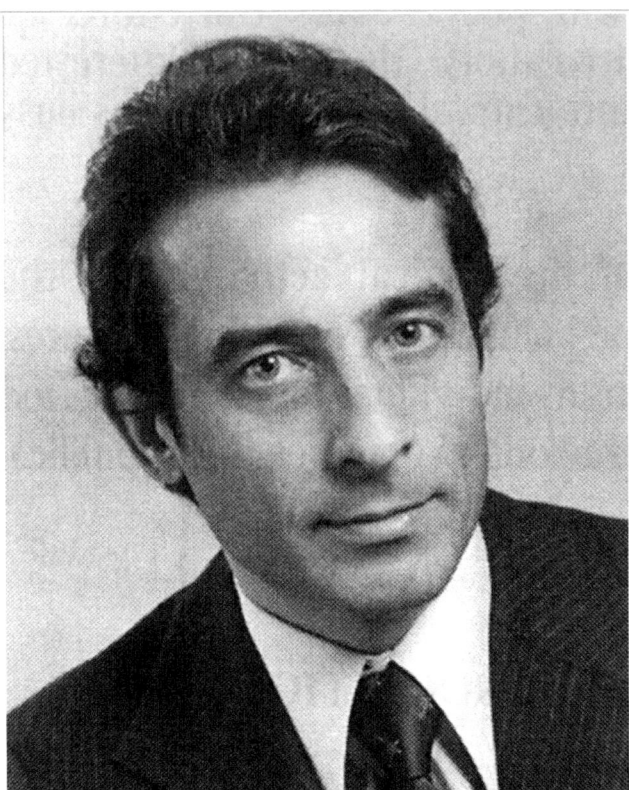
Erich Mühe

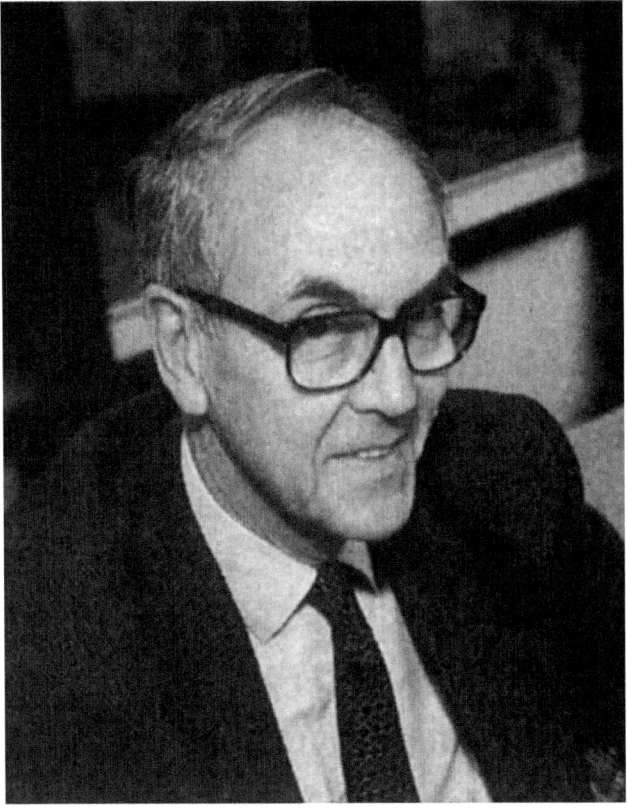
Francois Dubois

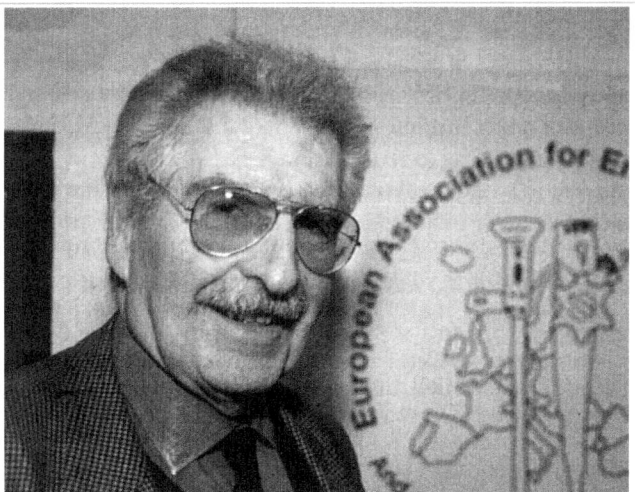

Jacques Perrisat

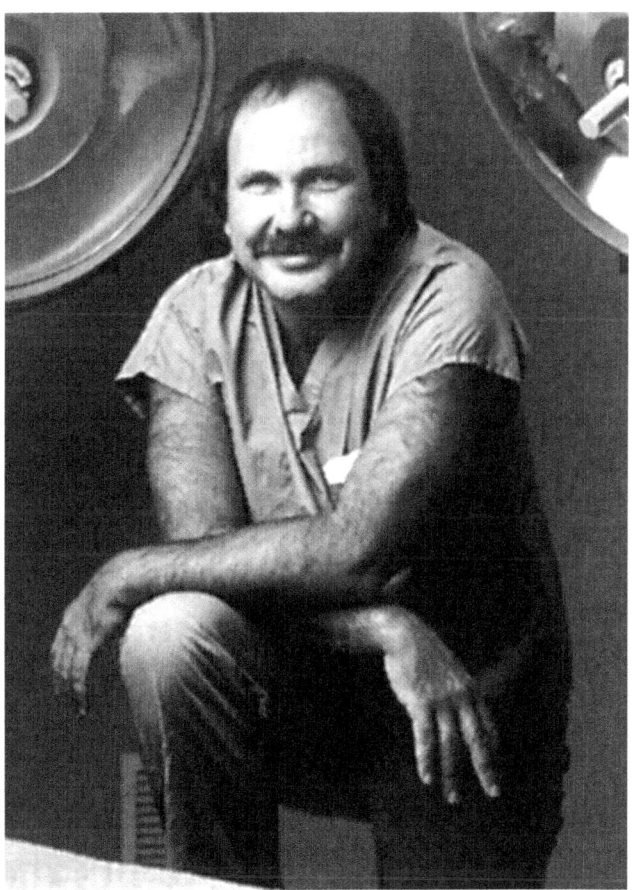

Eddie J. Reddick

Erich Mühe (1938–2005), a professional bike rider, developed a bed bike system for patients in the hospital to decrease postoperative pulmonary embolism. He developed a Galloscope, which was similar to a proctoscope in diameter. He created a small incision above the gallbladder for this large open tube system through which a light and, later, a telescope were introduced. His idea was not accepted and so he replaced the Galloscope with a laparoscope in 1987. Unfortunately, Mühe was killed in a bike accident in 2005 [1].

François Dubois (1930–) published the first laparoscopic cholecystectomy through celioscopie in *La Presse Médicale* in 1989 and followed with other laparoscopic cholecystectomy publications [2].

Jacques Perrisat (1923–) developed this procedure in 1989 in Bordeaux France. He published a year later his experience of laparoscopic cholecystectomies (1990). He made a major contribution to American surgeons when he appeared at the SAGES Board meeting in October 1989 in Louisville, Kentucky. He brought a videotape and requested a time spot for a demonstration. It was one of the major turning points to recognize a new procedure and its potential. It created a great debate at SAGES level and steps were taken to evaluate a new procedure [3].

Eddie J. Reddick (1949–2020) from Nashville, Tennessee, along with Douglas Olsen, performed their first cholecystectomy in September 1988. His group used an energy laser as a dissector for transection of the tissues and published their first initial experience in a laser journal followed a year later in the SAGES Journal, *Surgical Endoscopy* [4].

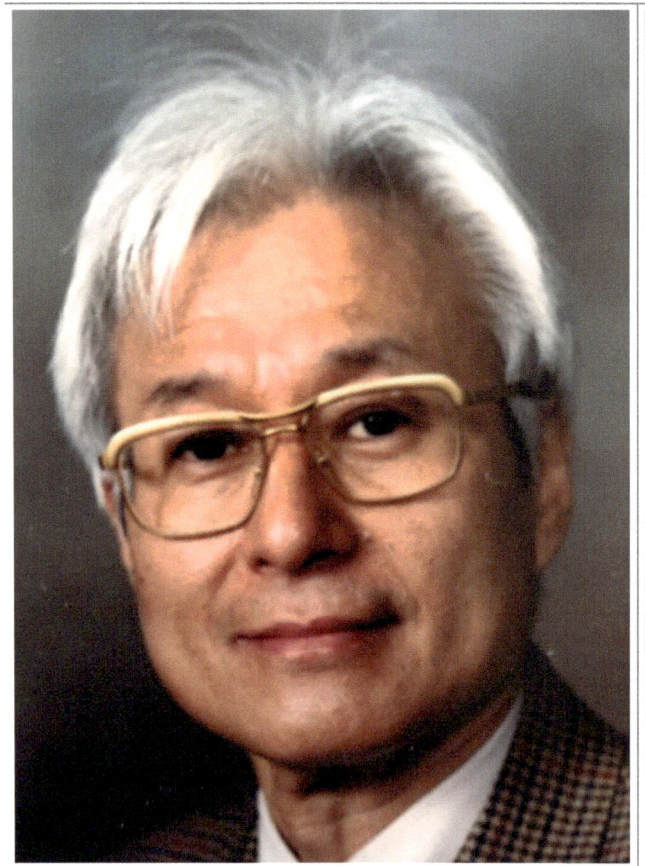

Sung Tao Ko

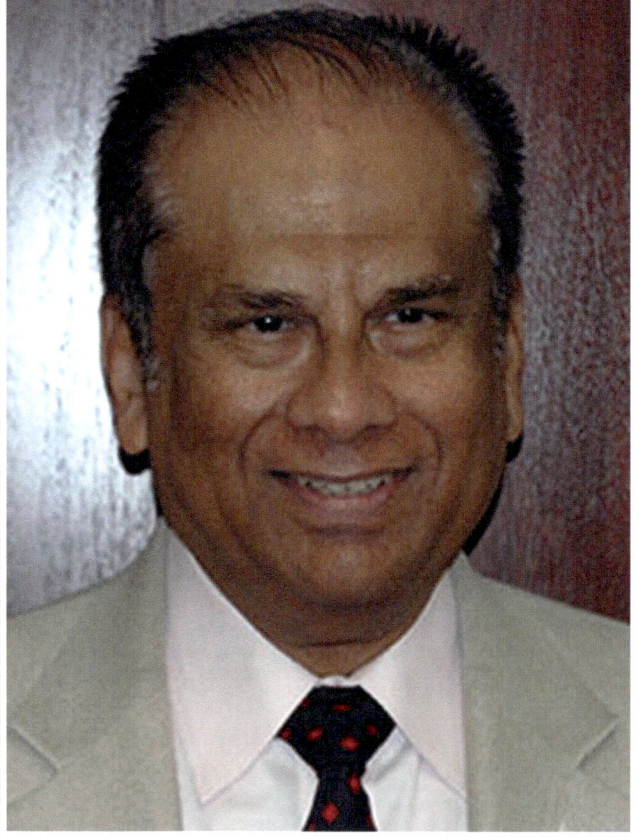

Mohan C. Airan

Doctors Ko and Airan published their first laparoscopic cholecystectomies in 1989, using a telescope with a teaching attachment for the assistant (no video) [5].

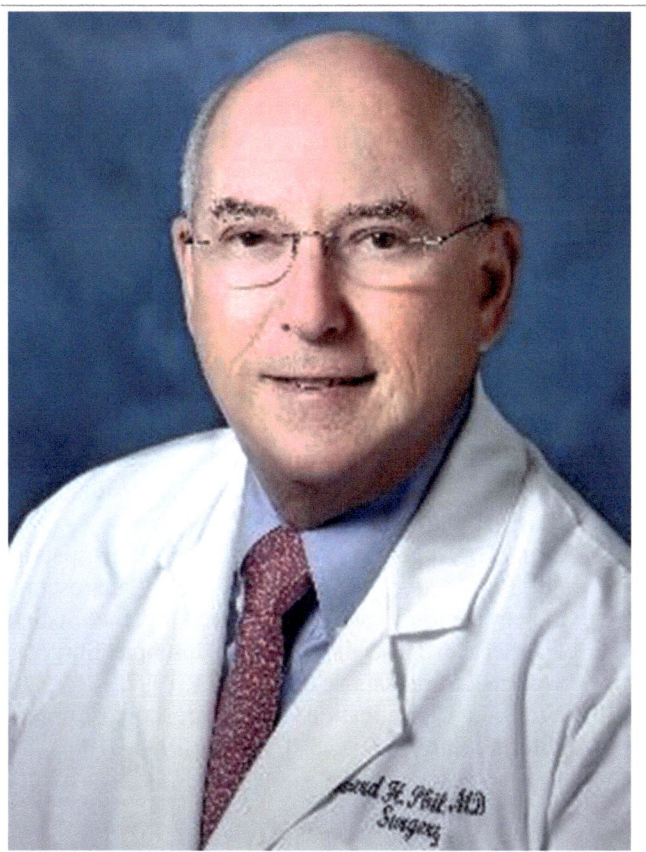

Edward H. Phillips

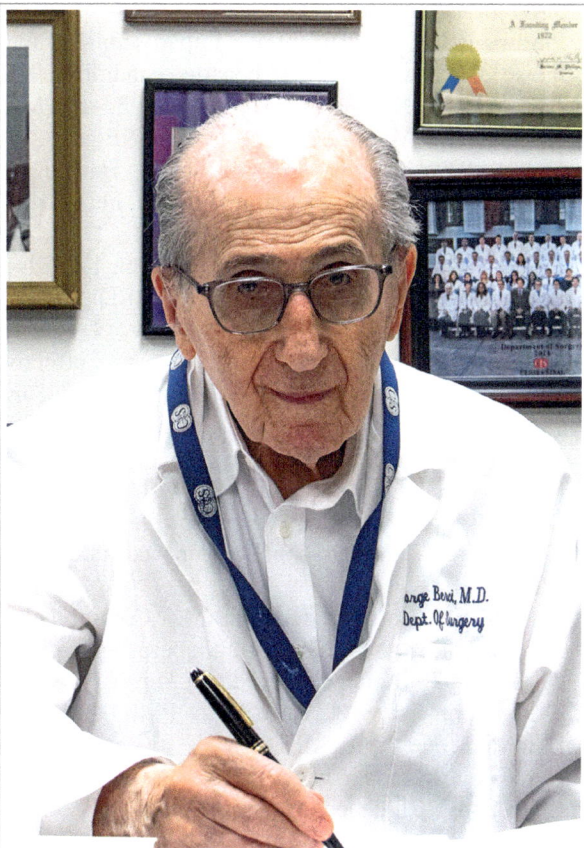

George Berci

Edward Phillips [6–14] and George Berci [15–23] visited Dubois in Paris and Reddick in the United States in early 1989. In May of the same year, they received the first laparoscopic sets and video system enabling them to begin work in the research lab before performing their first laparoscopic cholecystectomy in 1989 on patients. They published results of successful cases in 1989–1990.

References

1. Erich Mühe; A surgeon ahead of his time. Litynski G., History of Laparoscopy, page 87, Bernat Verlag, Frankfurt, 1996.
2. Dubois, F, Berthelot, G., Levard, H: Cholécystectomie par cœlioscopie, La Presse Méd. 18: 980–982 (1989)
3. Perrisat, J. Collet, D.: Belliard, R., Gallstones: Laparoscopic treatment – cholecystectomy, cholecystostomy, and lithotripsy. Our own experience. Surg Endosc. 4:1–5 (1990)
4. Reddick, EJ., Olsen, DO.: Laparoscopic laser cholecystectomy. A comparison with min-lap cholecystectomy. Surg Endosc 3: 131–133 (1989).
5. Ko, ST, Airan, MC, Early experience of Laparoscopic cholecystectomy, Chicago Surg. Soc. Scientific Program, Dec.1989
6. Phillips EH, Berci G, Carroll BJ, Daykhovsky L, Sackier J, Fallas MJ, Paz-Partlow M. "The importance of intraoperative cholangiography during laparoscopic cholecystectomy". *Am Surg*. 1990 Dec.: 56(12): 792–5. PMID 2148466 [PubMed-indexed for MEDLINE].
7. Sackier J, Berci G, Phillips E, Carroll B, Shapiro S, Paz-Partlow, M. "The role of cholangiography in laparoscopic cholecystectomy". *Arch Surg* 1991 Aug.: 126(8):1021–6. PMID 1830737 [PubMed-indexed for MEDLINE].
8. Phillips EH, Carroll BJ, Bello JM, Fallas MJ. "Laparoscopic cholecystectomy in acute cholecys-

titis", *Am Surg.* 1992 May: 58(5): 273–6. PMID 1535763 [PubMed-indexed for MEDLINE].
9. Carroll BJ, Phillips EH, Semel CJ, Fallas MJ, Morgenstern L. "Laparoscopic splenectomy". *Surgical Endoscopy.* 1992 July: 6(4): 183–5.
10. Phillips EH, Carroll BJ, et al. "Laparoscopic-guided biopsy for diagnosis of hepatic candidiasis". *J Laparoscopic Surgery.* 1992 Feb.: 2(1): 33–8. PMID 1533547 [PubMed-indexed for MEDLINE].
11. Carroll BJ, Chandra M, Phillips EH, Harold JG. "Laparoscopic cholecystectomy in the heart transplant candidate with acute cholecystitis". *J Heart Lung Transplant.* 1992 July-Aug.: 11(4 pt. 1): 831–3. PMID 1386754 [PubMed-indexed for MEDLINE].
12. Carroll BJ, Phillips EH, Daykhovsky L, et al. "Laparoscopic choledochoscopy: an effective approach to the common duct". *J Laparoscopic Surg.* 1992 Feb.: 2(1): 15–21. PMID 1533544 [PubMed-indexed for MEDLINE].
13. Phillips EH, Franklin MJ, Carroll BJ, et al, "Laparoscopic colectomy". *Ann Surg.* 1992 Dec.: 216(6): 703–7. PMID 1466626 [PubMed-indexed for MEDLINE].
14. Phillips EH, Carroll BJ, Fallas M. "Common duct stones: removal before or during laparoscopic cholecystectomy?" [Letter to the editor] *Surg Endoscopy.* 1992 Sept.-Oct.: 6(5): 266–8. PMID 1465739 [PubMed-indexed for MEDLINE].
15. Berci, G., Intraoperative and Postoperative Biliary Endoscopy (Choledochoscopy), Endoscopy 21:299-384, 1989.
16. Cuschieri, A., Berci, G. and McSherry, C., Laparoscopic Cholecystectomy (Editorial), Am J Surg 159:273–274, 1990.
17. Berci, G., Sackier, J. and Paz-Partlow, M., Laparoscopic Cholecystectomy Mini Access Surgery: Reality or Utopia?, Postgraduate General Surgery 2:50–54, 1990.
18. Phillips, E., Berci, G., Carroll, B., et al., The Importance of Intraoperative Cholangiography during Laparoscopic Cholecystectomy, Am J Surg, 56:792–795, 1990.
19. Sackier, J., Berci, G. and Paz-Partlow, M., Laparoscopic Transcystic Choledocholithotomy as an Adjunct to Laparoscopic Cholecystectomy., Am J Surg 571: 323–329, 1991
20. Berci, G., Sackier, J. and Paz Partlow, M., New Ideas and Improved Instrumentation for Laparoscopic Cholecystectomy, Surg Endosc 5: 1–4, 1991.
21. Berci, G., Cholangiography and Choledochoscopy During Laparoscopic Cholecystectomy, Its Place and Value, Dig Surg 8: 92–96, 1991.
22. Airan, M., Appel, M., Berci, G., et al., Retrospective and Prospective Multi-Institutional Laparoscopic Cholecystectomy Study Organized by the Society of American Gastrointestinal Endoscopic Surgeons (SAGES), Surg Endosc 6: 169–177, 1992.
23. Berci, G., Complications of Laparoscopic Surgery, Editorial, Surg Endosc 8: 165–166, 1994.

Cholangiography in the Operating Room

J. Andrew Hamlin

Abstract

Cholangiography performed during biliary surgery provides the surgeon with valuable information regarding the anatomy of the biliary tree and potential presence of ductal calculi. Progress in the technical accomplishment of this radiographic contribution to surgery, fluorocholangiography, has contributed to improved statistics regarding ductal injuries and retained calculi.

Keywords

Intraoperative cholangiography · Fluorocholangiography · Biliary imaging

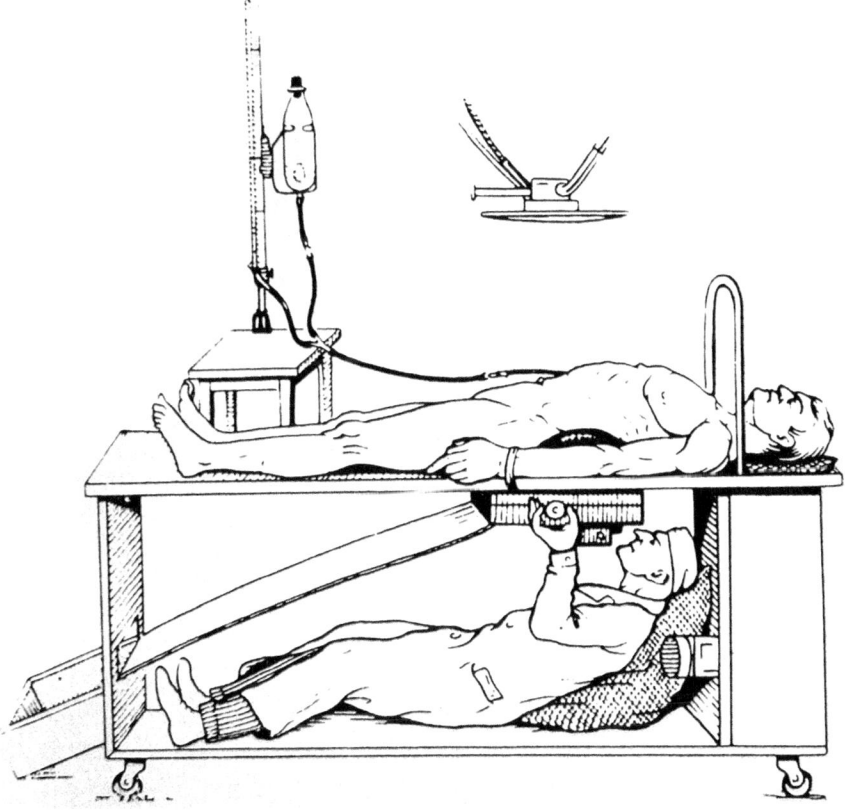

It was recommended to design an operating room table which incorporates a fluoroscopic screen with a radiologist in supine position during the biliary operation. (Porscher and Caroli, 1955)

The original version of this chapter was revised. The correction to this chapter can be found at https://doi.org/10.1007/978-3-030-76845-4_20

The first radiographic report of biliary ductal opacification was in 1915. Through an unsuspected communication between the duodenum and gallbladder, barium, given for an upper GI series, was seen to opacify the biliary tree. Subsequently, abdominal cutaneous fistulography also provided a route for opaque material to gain entrance to the biliary tree. Radiographic demonstration of the bile ducts occurred serendipitously when a mixture of petrolatum paste and bismuth was introduced into a cutaneous fistula that developed in a female patient that had undergone pelvic surgery 2 years earlier [1]. Lipiodol, an oil-based agent, temporarily replaced bismuth as the contrast agent of choice [2]. However, because of the physical properties of the oil, water-soluble iodinated agents came to be preferred over lipiodol. In 1929, using a two-staged surgical approach for patients with acute cholecystitis or cholangitis, Cotte recommended placing a decompression tube in the gallbladder or common duct and examining the biliary tree by injecting contrast material through the indwelling tube prior to the second operation [3].

Intraoperative cholangiography was introduced in the early 1930s by Mirizzi and Losada [4, 5]. It was readily apparent, using their technique, that the bile duct anatomy, as well as any ductal leaks and possibly intraductal calculi could be appreciated and dealt with prior to closing the incision. While radiographic equipment improved from that time until the late 1970s, the basic technique of intraoperative cholangiography remained largely unchanged. This rather cumbersome technique may account for the low percentage of biliary surgeons that adopted it.

Standard Operative Cholangiography [6]

At the appropriate moment, when surgical exposure permitted, the surgeon placed a small catheter or metal cannula into either the cystic duct or the extrahepatic bile duct (Fig. 14.1). A syringe con-

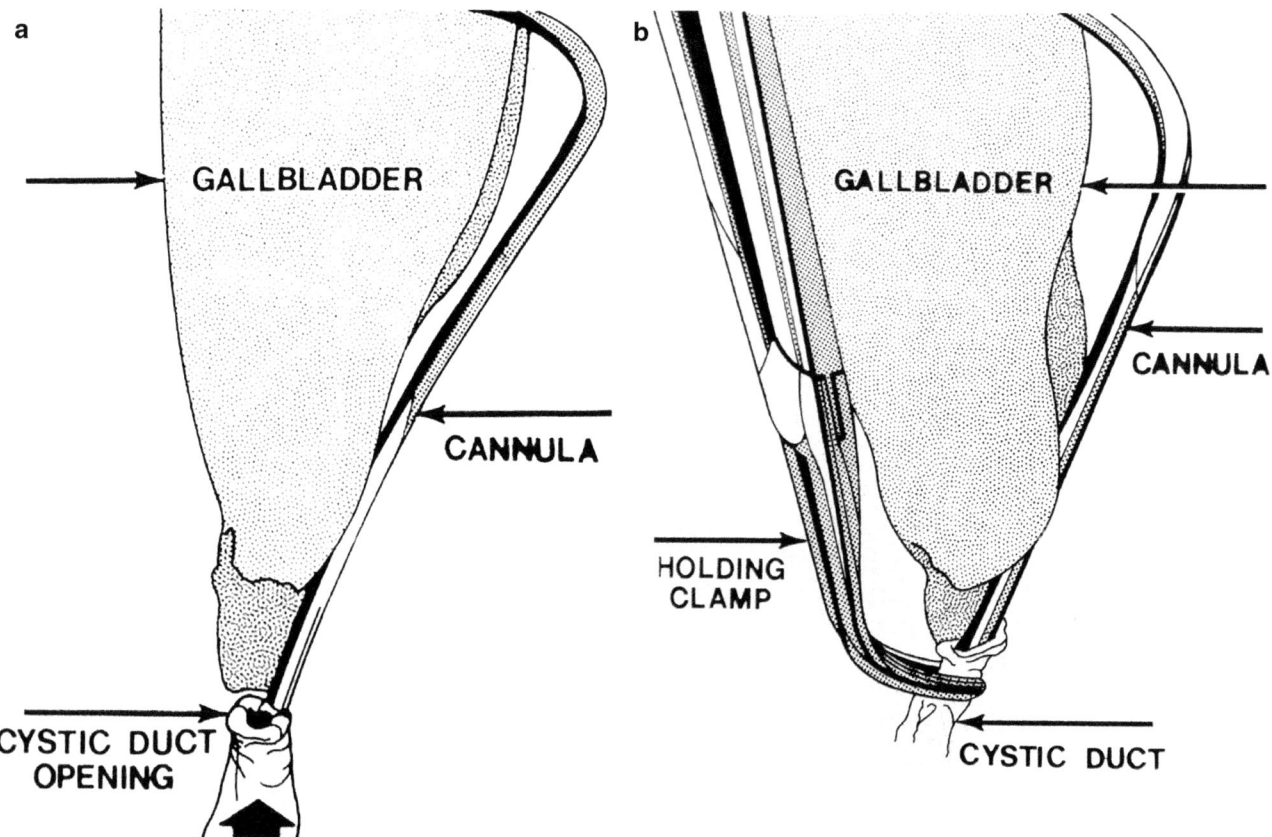

Fig. 14.1 (a) Injection cannula directed toward the opened cystic duct. (b) The cannula has been secured in the cystic duct by a holding clamp

taining radiographic contrast material was attached by extension tubing to the catheter/cannula and a sterile drape was placed over the incision. The x-ray technician, standing by, was summoned.

The patient was rolled slightly to the left in order for the x-ray technician to place a radiographic film cassette between the patient and the operating table, corresponding to the location of the liver and bile ducts. Next the patient was rolled slightly to the right to avoid having the extrahepatic duct projected on the spine. A portable x-ray machine was either brought into the operating room (OR) and rolled to the side of the operating table. The x-ray tube was then positioned.

The surgeon began to slowly inject 2–3 ml of contrast material and tell the x-ray technician when to make an exposure. This process was commonly repeated twice with additional small quantities of contrast material injected for each exposure. The x-ray technician then took the three film cassettes to the dark room to be processed. Ten to fifteen minutes would elapse before he/she would return to the OR with the developed images. The total time required was approximately 20–30 minutes.

Operative Fluoro-Cholangiography

In 1948, Porcher and Caroli [8] suggested designing an operating table with an overhead x-ray tube and a fluoroscopic screen attached underneath that could be viewed by a radiologist lying beneath the table. The impracticality of this arrangement failed to generate interest.

Through the 1950s and 1960s progressive development of fluoroscopic image intensification along with improvement in television display made possible real time observation of high-quality images. With development of portable image intensification, various investigators [7, 9–12] began to employ the equipment in the OR for cholangiography and it also became an important tool for orthopedic surgery. By the mid-1970s, these improvements were incorporated in a portable C-arm apparatus. The C-arm construction assured the alignment of the x-ray beam with the image intensifier (Fig. 14.2).

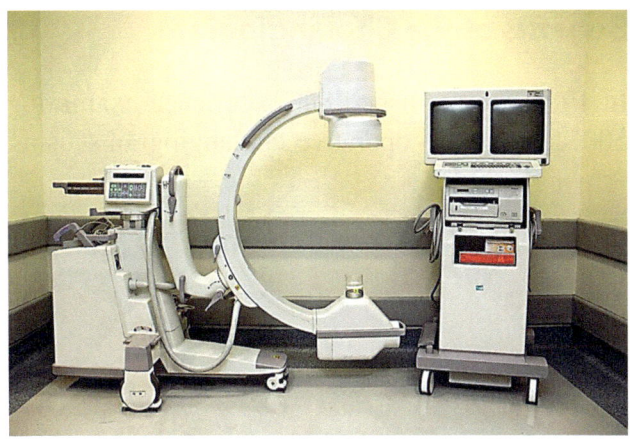

Fig. 14.2 Portable C-arm for fluoroscopy with accompanying mobile imaging screens and recording apparatus

For use in the OR, particularly in operative cholangiography, a brief fluoroscopic exposure displayed on the television monitor makes it easy to be certain the biliary tree is in the field of view. If not, the technician could make the necessary positioning adjustments. Before injecting diluted water-soluble contrast material, a short fluoroscopic image and scout exposure of the surgical field would also alert the surgeon to the presence of opaque objects such as hemoclips, instruments, retractors, monitoring wires, nasogastric tubes, or sponge markers that might obscure the ducts. If possible, these opaque objects should be removed from the field. During the study, the televised images are viewed in real time by the operating surgeon and 6–8 permanent images, captured from the image intensifier, are exposed and stored. With remote audio-visual connection to the x-ray department, the participating radiologist simultaneously views the television images and can communicate with the surgeon.

It became apparent that the use of undiluted iodinated contrast material could obscure ductal calculi, therefore water-soluble contrast material (diatrizoate: Renografin-60 or Hypaque), diluted 50–50 with saline, was preferred (Fig. 14.3). With a slow, progressive injection of the diluted contrast material, a gradual increase in opacification of the ducts also improved diagnostic accuracy (Fig. 14.4). For a permanent record, individual images could be exposed as the study progressed. Cholangiography requires approximately 10–15 minutes.

Benefits of the Cholangiogram

In 1981, we published our experience examining 500 consecutive operative cholangiograms using the fluorocholangiographic method (6–9 films per patient) [13].

Biliary Ductal Anatomy

Variations from the standard anatomy of both the segmental intrahepatic and extrahepatic bile ducts are common. A cholangiogram presents a map of the ducts and knowledge of that display may prevent a ductal injury to one or more of these anatomies.

The usual anatomic display shows the right dorsocaudal segmental duct joining the right ventrocranial segmental duct to form the right hepatic duct. In our material that anatomical relationship occurred only 72% of the time. In 22%, the right dorsocaudal segmental duct joined the left hepatic duct. The right ventrocranial segmental duct joined the left hepatic duct while the right dorsocaudal branch continued as the right hepatic duct in 6%.

The confluence of the right and left hepatic ducts forms the common hepatic duct, the length of which may vary depending on the level of confluence of the hepatic ducts. Also, occasionally noted are accessory ducts, usually small, which

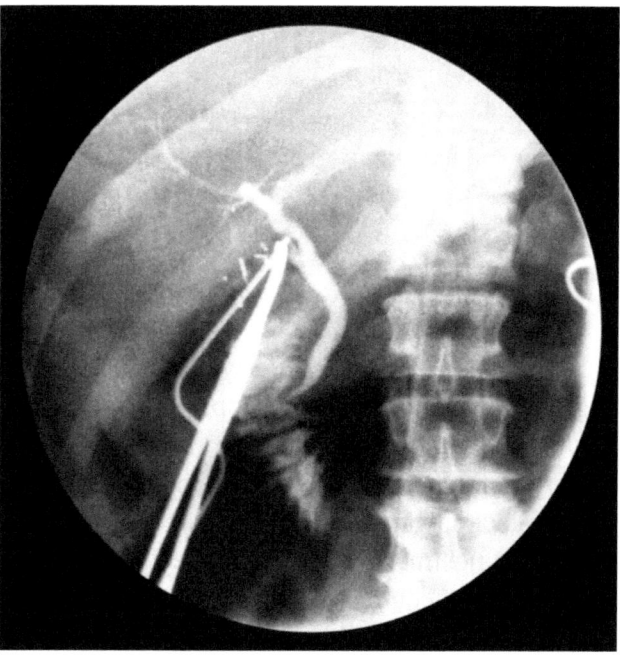

Fig. 14.3 Bile duct opacification, including the sphincteric portion, with contrast material flowing into the duodenum. Note the cannula, holding clamp and hemoclip

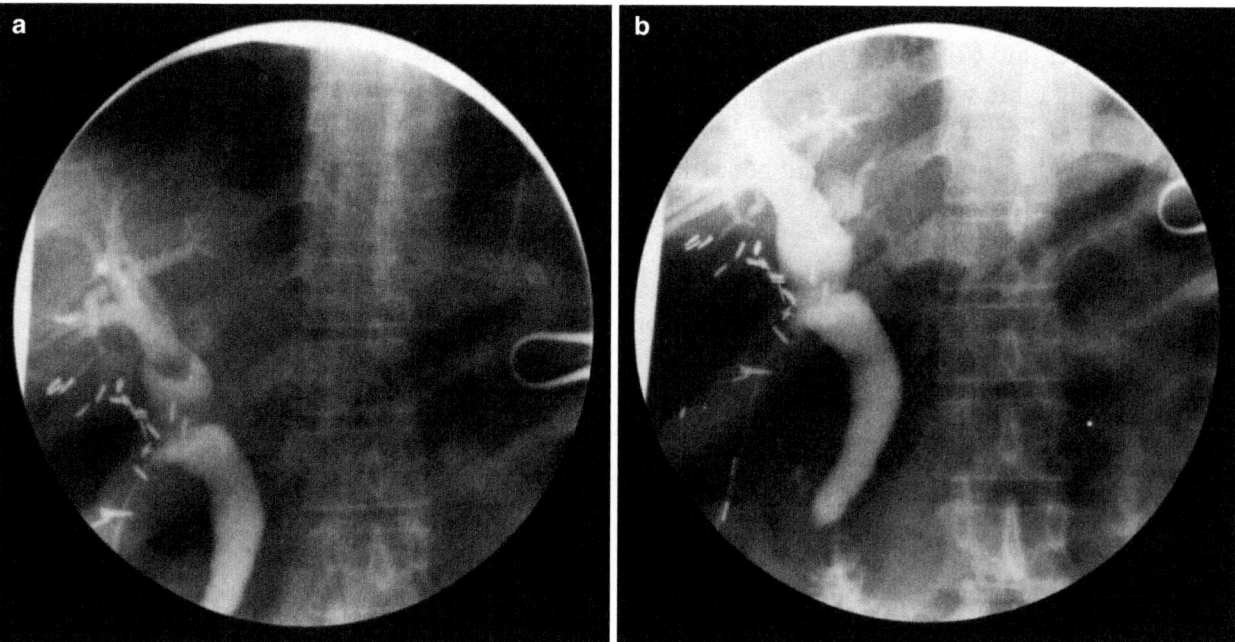

Fig. 14.4 Calculi may be obscured by contrast material that is either too dense or over-injected. (**a**) Faceted calculus is shown in the common hepatic duct. (**b**) With additional contrast injected the calculus is obscured

Biliary Duct Stones

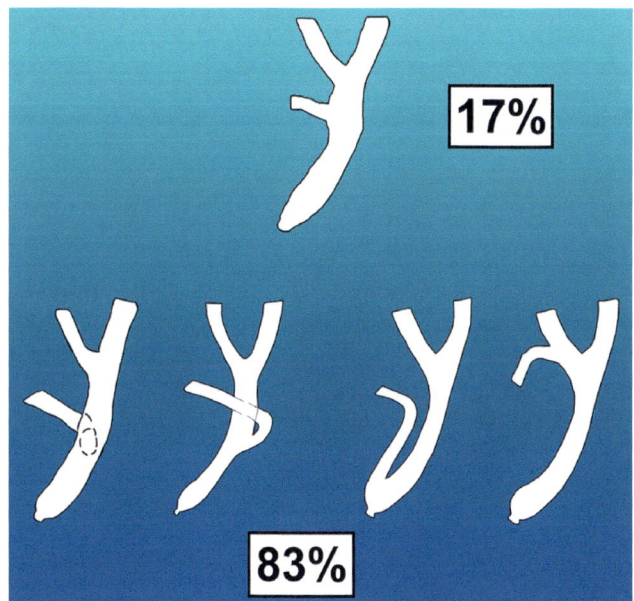

Fig. 14.5 Cystic duct anatomy. The lateral entry is only 17%. Anterior or posterior entry: 41%. Spiral type: 35% and a parallel run: 7%. The recognition of the cystic duct anatomy at an early part of surgery (by IOC) is of great help to recognize injuries in time

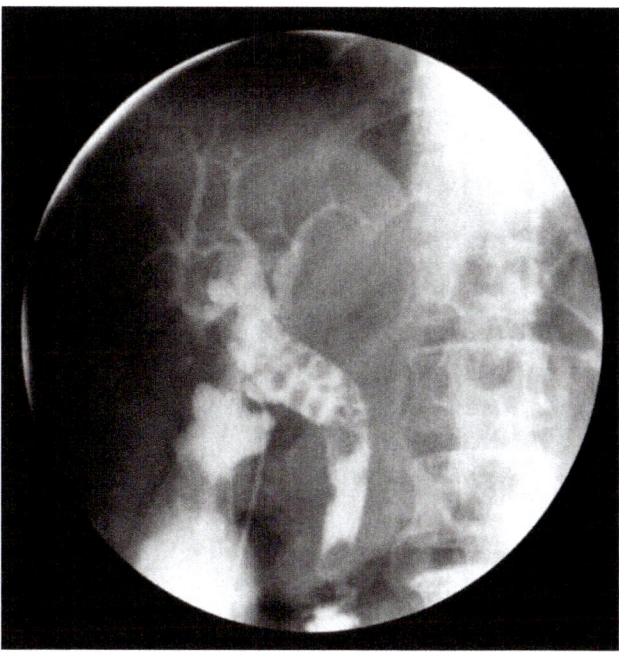

Fig. 14.6 Common hepatic duct calculus is demonstrated. When numerous ductal calculi are discovered, making complete clearing difficult or impossible, a choledochoduodenostomy may be necessary

exit the liver and join the common hepatic duct. When these variations or anomalies occur unexpectedly, the potential for transection leading to postoperative bile leak is great.

In most textbooks the cystic duct is usually shown entering the lateral aspect of the extrahepatic common duct. In our study, that occurred in only 17% of cases. In 41% of our cases, the entry was either anteriorly or posteriorly into the common duct, while a spiral course of the cystic duct was noted in 35% with the cystic duct passing posterior to the common duct to enter on the medial aspect of the common duct (Fig. 14.5). In 7%, the cystic duct coursed parallel to the common bile duct on its lateral aspect to join it near the sphincter.

Biliary Duct Stones

When the clinical presentation suggests the presence of choledocholithiasis, cholangiography and common duct exploration are expected (Fig. 14.6). In many patients that present for cholecystectomy, however, no signs or symptoms of choledocholithiasis were recognized prior to surgery. In our experience with 500 consecutive cholecystectomies, each of which underwent routine operative fluorocholangiograms, we found unsuspected calculi in 25 patients. Five percent of our patients had unsuspected ductal calculi that were discovered on the operative fluorocholangiogram, each of which had the stones removed during the primary operation, thereby obviating the need for a subsequent operation. Our findings concur with other investigators that have reported unsuspected ductal calculi in 4–10% of patients (Figs. 14.7 and 14.8).

In open surgery (choledochotomy) the surgeon is placing a T-tube and performing a completion cholangiography to make sure no stones were left. In approximately 3–4 weeks (with no symptoms) a cholangiogram is made before the T-tube is pulled. In case an overlooked stone was found, we were able to remove it with local anesthesia with the help of the Choledochoscope (Fig. 14.9).

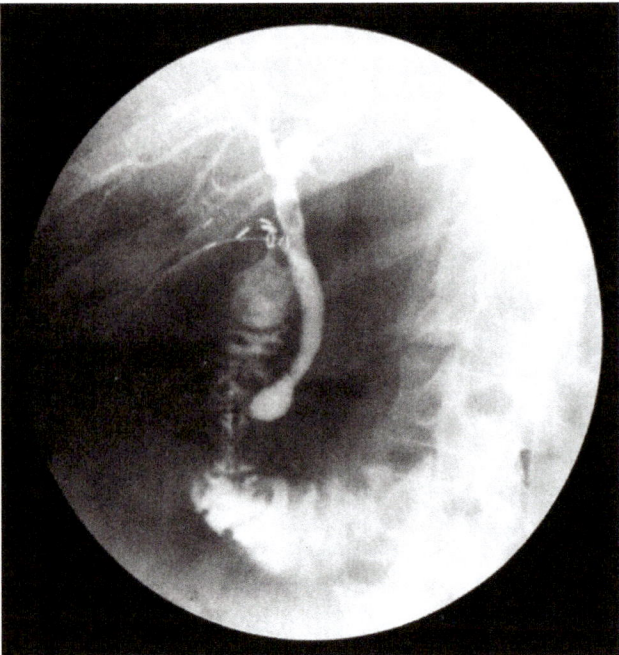

Fig. 14.7 Common hepatic duct calculus. Fusiform dilatation of the distal common duct

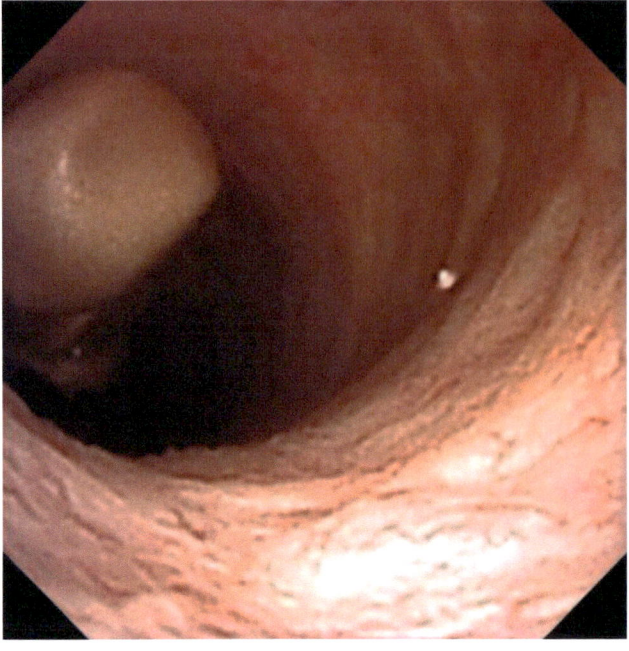

Fig. 14.9 Intraoperative Choledochoscopy is known. In certain cases of difficult anatomy, it is easy to remove them under visual control

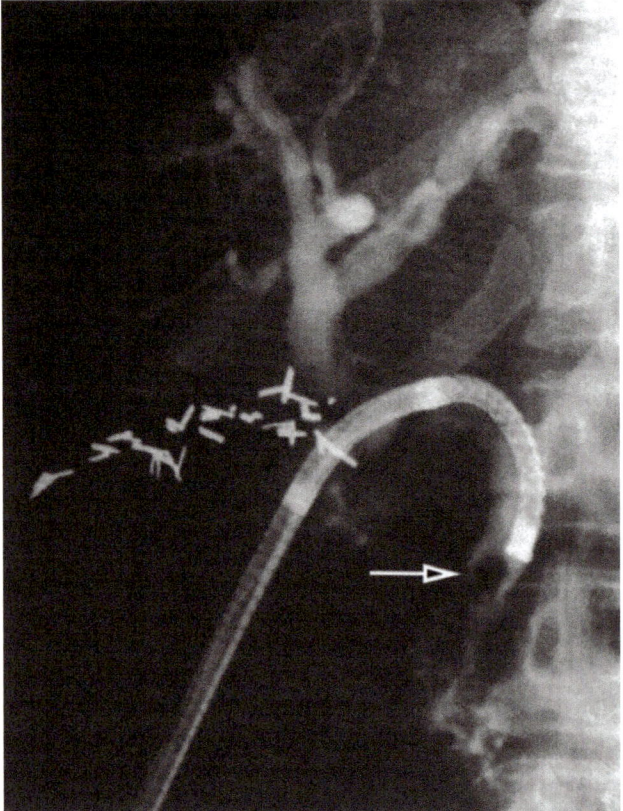

Fig. 14.8 Retained stone found in the T-tube tract which was removed with a choledochoscope through the T-tube during the postoperative period [14]

References

1. Carman RD: Roentgen observation of the gallbladder and hepatic ducts after perforation into duodenum. JAMA 65:1812, 1915.
2. Reich A: Accidental injection of bile ducts with petrolatum and bismuth paste. JAMA 71:1555, 1918.
3. Cotte MG: Exploration of the biliary ducts with lipiodol in a case of fistula. Bull Mem Soc Natl Chir (Paris) 23:759–767, 1925.
4. Cotte MG: Sur 1: Exploration radiologique des vies biliares avec injection lipiodol après cholecystectomie ou choledocotomie. Bull Mem Soc Natl Chir (Paris) 55:863,1929.
5. Mirizzi PL, Losada CQ: Exploration of the bile ducts during an operation. Proceedings of the Third Argentine Congress of Surgery. 1:694–703,1931.
6. Mirizzi PL: La cholangiographia durante las operaciones de las vias biliares. Bol soc cir Buenos Aires 16:1133, 1932.
7. Berci G, Shore JM, Hamlin JA, Morgenstern, L. Operative fluoroscopy and cholangiography. Am Surg 135:32, 1978.
8. Porcher P, Caroli J: Radiomanometrie biliare peroperatoire en controle radioscopique permanent. Inform. Sem. Hosp. 14:523, 1948.
9. Grace RH, Peckar VG: The value of operative cholangiography using an image intensifier and television monitor. Br J Surg 55:933, 1968.

References

10. Berci G, Steckel R: Modern radiology in the operating room. Arch Surg 197:577, 1973.
11. Berci G, Zheutlin N: Improving radiology in surgery. Med Instrum 10:110, 1976.
12. Berci G, Hamlin JA, Morgenstern L, Fisher DL: Modern operative fluorocholangiography. Gastrointest Radiol 3:401, 1978.
13. Berci G, Hamlin JA: Operative biliary radiology. Williams and Wilkins, Baltimore, 1981.
14. Berci G, Hamlin JA: A Combined Fluoroscopic and Endoscopic Approach for Retrieval of Retained Stones through the T-Tube Tract, Surg Gyn Obstet, 153: 237, 1987.

Bile Duct Injuries

Abstract

Operative cholangiograms performed during laparoscopic cholecystectomy may identify anomalies of the biliary system in order to reduce the incidence of ductal injury. The use of these techniques may disclose extravasation of contrast agents that indicate ductal injuries. Once identified, these injuries may be corrected if appropriate surgical skill sets are available.

Keywords

Bile duct injury · Bile duct anomalies · Operative cholangiography

Biliary surgery was well known to the practicing surgeons. The sudden introduction of a different procedure (laparoscopic) was new for the already trained surgeon to accept and then be re-trained.

Having experience and data collected in the past 15 years, it was logical to think that in a closed, technically more difficult, surgical procedure, the already-known IOC process would be of help and be accepted [1].

In case of unexpected anatomical findings and contrast leakage seen on IOC, the patient could be explored immediately, and more complex postoperative surgeries avoided.

Two major complications were observed: bile duct injuries (Fig. 15.1) and existing or retained CBD stones [2]. The problems were already reported in 1932 by Mirizzi [3] who recommended operative cholangiography, based on his experience.

In the organized tutorial sessions by SAGES (Society of American Gastrointestinal and Endoscopic Surgeons), IOC was included in the program but when it came to the transfer to their own practice, in the majority of cases, it was not performed.

The extension of OR time of 10–15 minutes, for example, in a 90–120-minute surgery, does not create complications.

The technician was called in at the start of cholangiography. The mobile image amplifier used also by orthopedic surgeons was brought in and placed on the patient's right side after the case is anesthetized. Additional tools and contrast materials are prepared by the nurse.

Surgeons, assistants, and nurses need lead aprons. There is no radiation hazard to the patient or the personnel [4] (Figs. 15.2 and 15.3).

After one or two cases of a training period, it takes approximately 15 minutes OR time extension to complete the procedure.

During slow injections, the anomalies of the cystic duct are immediately visible, and the entire (normal) anatomy of the Biliary tract (Figs. 15.4 and 15.5) are observed.

In case of operative cholangiograms, the most important findings, such as anomalies, extravasation of contrast or ductal injuries can be immediately recognized, and corrective surgery initiated

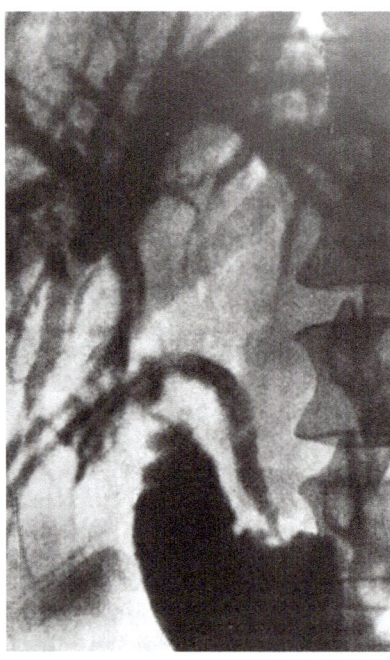

Fig. 15.1 Operative cholangiogram showing acute ductal injury

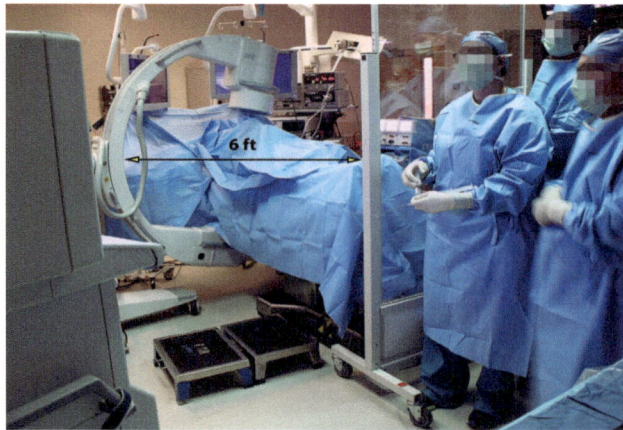

Fig. 15.3 The surgeon and the scrub nurse with a lead apron standing behind a mobile translucent lead shield. There will be almost zero hazard of radiation in case of 6 feet [4]

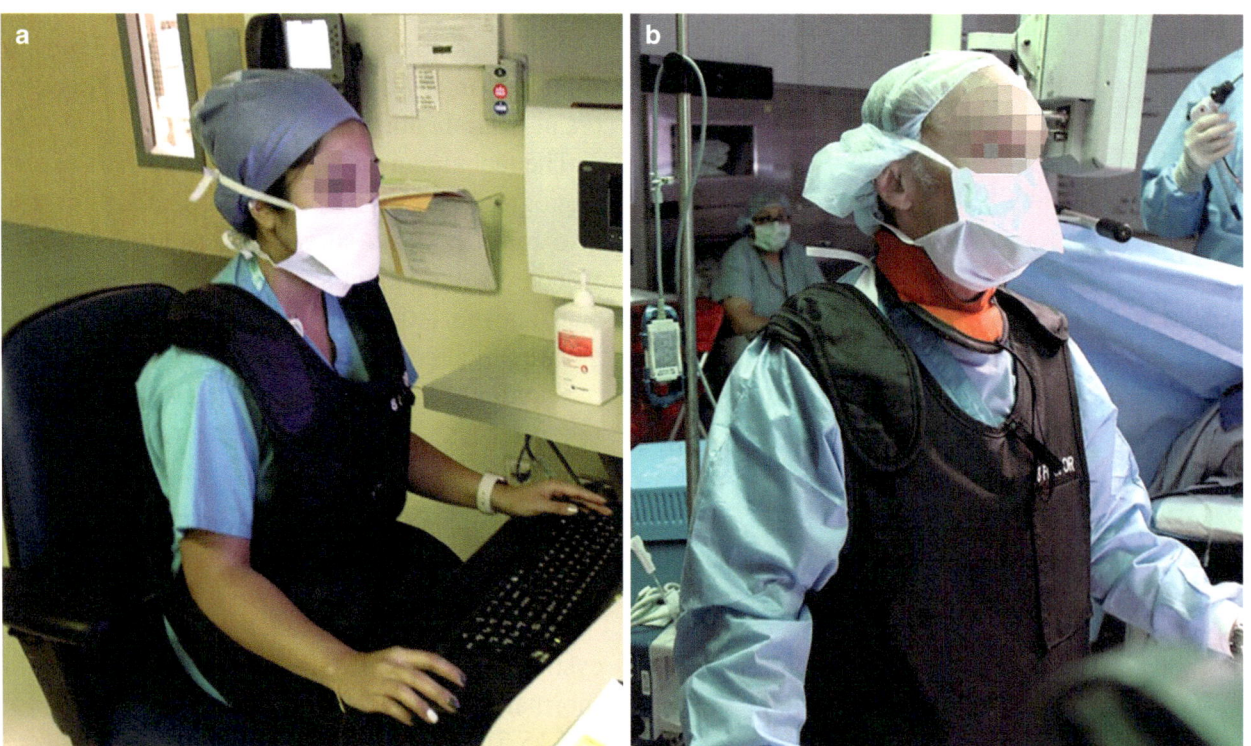

Fig. 15.2 Nurse and anesthesiologist should have a lead protective apron when performing an IOC

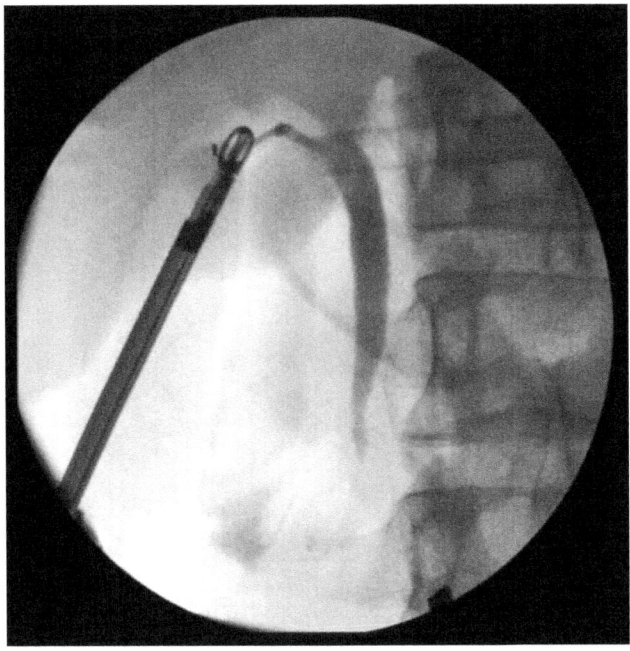

Fig. 15.4 A distal CBD with sphincter and the contrast

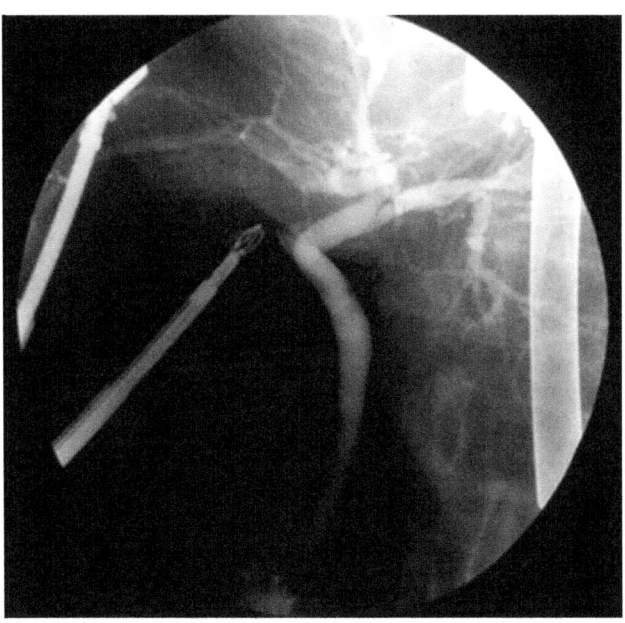

Fig. 15.6 Pulling a short cystic duct, the hepatic duct can be easily clipped

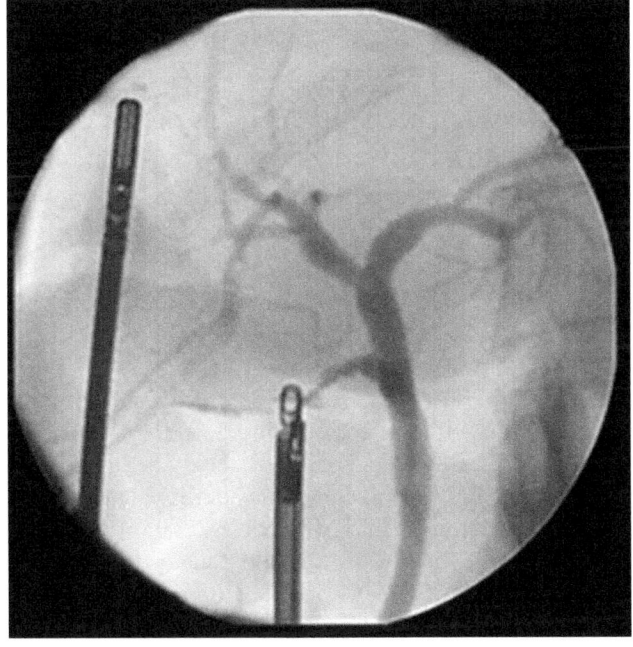

Fig. 15.5 The proximal hepatic system with branches is well-seen

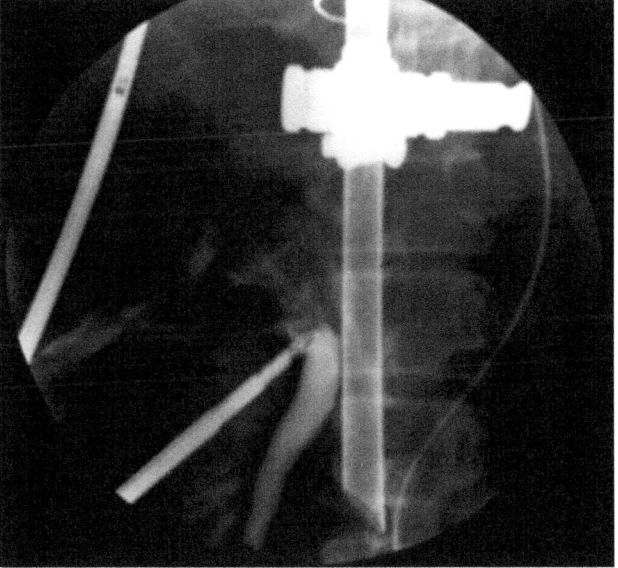

Fig. 15.7 This was a complete dissection of the CBD, which was immediately discovered and explored during the laparoscopic procedure. A Ductal-entero-anastomosis was performed in the first session. Followed up and no symptoms

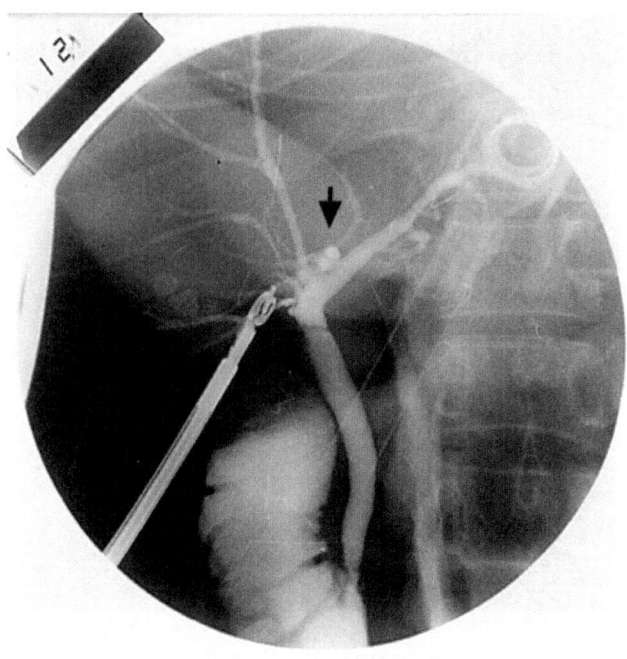

Fig. 15.8 Small extravasations were observed, and the patient was explored and repaired. The case was followed for several months without complications

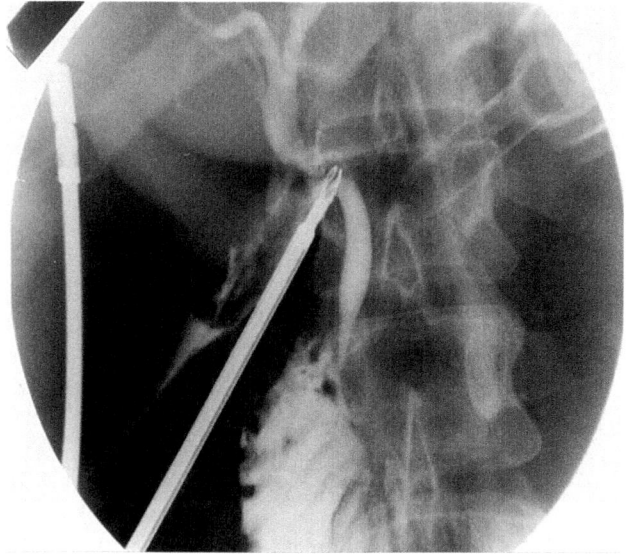

Fig. 15.9 Ductal injury immediately recognized and explored. Ductal continuity established and drained. Patient followed up to 3 months. No second surgery

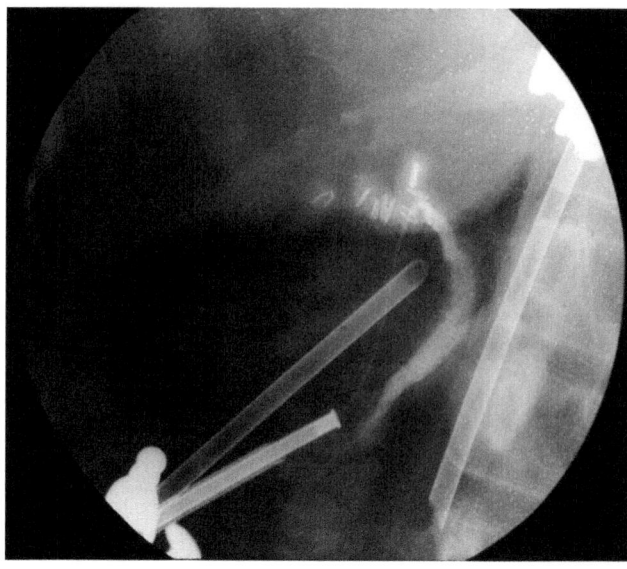

Fig. 15.10 During cholangiography, no contrast material was detected in the proximal duct, and therefore, the case was immediately explored, clips removed. It was possible to re-anastomoze the hepatic duct and evaluate the continuity by repeated cholangiograms. Followed up for 3 months. No symptoms

(Figs. 15.6, 15.7, 15.8, 15.9, and 15.10). The patient does not need to wait with symptoms to be referred with an acute abdomen for re-exploration with a high morbidity and mortality.

References

1. Hamlin, JA. Critical analysis, Chapter 17. In: Berci G, Hamlin, JA, editors. Operative biliary radiology. Baltimore: Williams and Wilkins; 1981.
2. Phillips, E., Berci, G., Carroll, B., et al The importance of intraoperative cholangiography during Laparoscopic Cholecystectomy, Am J Surg 56: 792–795, 1990.
3. Mirizzi PL., La Cholangiografia durante las Operaciones de las vias Biliares. Bol. Soc Cir Buenos Aires. 1932; 6:1133, pages 5–9.
4. Donna Early, Chapter 4: Radiation Hazard in Berci, G. Hamlin JA. Operative Biliary Radiology. Baltimore: Williams & Wilkins, 1981, p. 23–38.

Common Bile Duct Stones and Choledocholithotomy

Abstract

The presence of CBD stones occurs in 70,000–100,000 (10%) cholecystectomies per year. The video choledochoscope made it easier to discover these calculi and to remove extrahepatic stones during the initial operation. Appropriate teaching of surgical stone extraction at the time of laparoscopic cholecystectomy is lacking in academic medical centers leading to greater dependence on postoperative ERCP.

Keywords

Common bile duct stones · Endoscopic stone extraction · Retained stones

The removal of a stone(s) during an open common bile exploration was sometimes a difficult task due to the variety of the anatomy, inflammations, size and location of calculi, just to mention a few factors. The introduction of IOC was a great help. Endoscopic inspection of the anatomy therefore was improved. The incidents of retained calculi decreased [1].

The video choledochoscope made it easier to discover the calculi, to see the anatomy, the anomalies, the stone, and the basket position on an enlarged screen and obtain help from the assistant and scrub nurse [2]. It became a significant helping factor during laparoscopic lithotomy to complete the entire procedure in one session [3] (Figs. 16.1, 16.2, and 16.3).

CBD Stones

The presence of CBD stones occurs in 70,000–100,000 cases per year. The successful removal of CBD stones during laparoscopy is well known and has been done with the help of IOC by trained surgeons combining CBD stone removal with IOC and choledochoscopy in the same session (Table 16.1). Today, 700,000 patients have to undergo a second procedure with 5% pancreatitis and 1 to 2 days hospitalization or 0.1–0.2% of perforation or bleeding requiring urgent intervention [4–14].

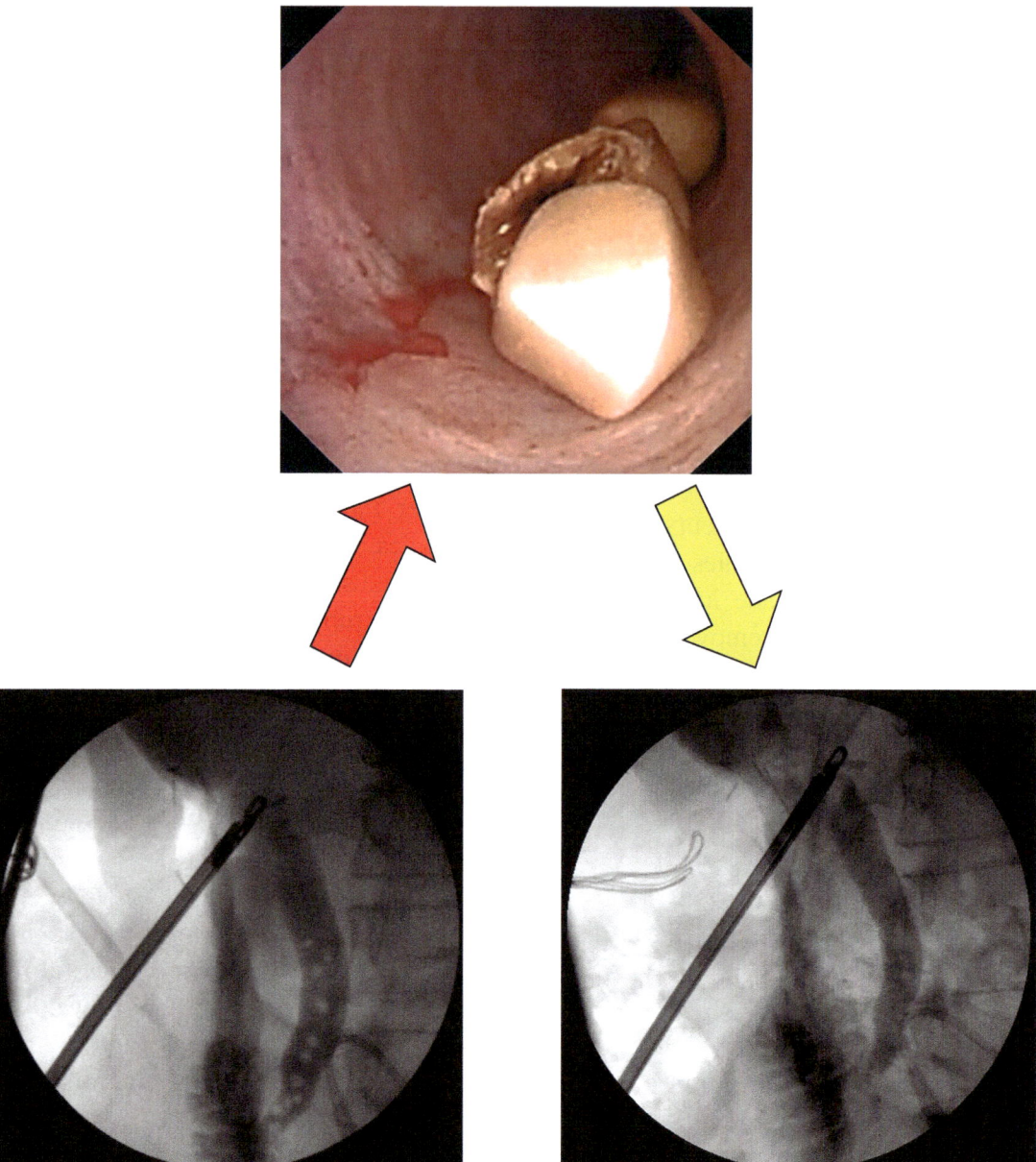

Figs. 16.1, 16.2, 16.3 Removal of CBD stones in ONE session. Choledochoscope and Cholangiogram show Multiple stones. No stones in the distal duct on completion cholangiogram

Table 16.1 Results of laparoscopic biliary surgery from the Department of Surgery, Cedars Sinai Medical Center

Laparoscopic Cholecystectomies 2014–2020	
Laparoscopic Cholecystectomy	663
Intraoperative cholangiography	663
CBD stones	60

We would like to acknowledge the Cedars Sinai Medical Center surgeons who performed IOC, the surgery and reported their findings: Matthew B. Bloom, MD, FACS, Miguel A. Burch, MD, FACS, Brendon J. Carroll, MD, FACS, David E. Fermelia, MD, FACS, Neel R. Joshi, MD, FACS, Edwards H. Phillips, MD, FACS, and Gregory K. Tsushima, MD, FACS.

Figures 16.1 and 16.2 demonstrate CBD stones removed by choledochoscopy, and Fig. 16.3 shows a final negative cholangiogram of the CBD system.

Improved visual removal of calculi (Surgeon, assistant, and nurse can see the enlarged image)

(a) Large stone in the CBD.

(b) Impacted stone near the sphincter area.

(c) Precise position and entrapment of stone by the basket.

(d) The hepatic ductal system can be also inspected.

References

Publications

1. Phillips, E., Berci, G., et al., The Role of Choledochoscopy: The eternal problem of how to remove a CBD stone, J. Surgical Innovation, 22:540–545, 2015.
2. Laparoscopic cholecystectomy: first, do no harm; second, take care of bile duct stones. Berci, G., Hunter, J., Morgenstern, L., Arregui, M. et al., Surg Endosc 27: 1051–1054, 2013.
3. Santos, F., Soper, N., Choledocholithiasis, Springer 2018, Chann, Switzerland.

ERCP USA

4. Prospective Randomized Trial of LC + LCBDE vs ERCP/S + LC for Common Bile Duct Stone Disease., Rogers, Stanley et al, Arch Surg, 2010, 145 (1): 28–33
5. Complications of ERCP, ASGE Standards of Practical Committee, Gie, 2012, 75(3): 467–470
6. Surgeon, ERCP and Laparoscopic Common Bile Duct Exploration: do we need a standard approach for Common Bile Duct Stones., Baucom, RB et al., Surg Endosc, 2016, 30: 414–423
7. Algorithm for the management of ERCP-Related perforations., Kumbhari, V., Gastrointestinal Endoscopy, 2016, 83(5): 934–943
8. Predictive Risk Factors Associated with Cholangitis following ERCP., Tierney, J., Bhutiani, N., Stamp, B., Richey, JS., Bahr, MH, Vitale, GC., Surg Endosc, 2018, 32: 799–804

ERCP International

9. Laparoscopic transcystic exploration for single-stage management of common duct stones and acute cholecystitis., Chirurgia, M. et al, Surg Endosc, 2012, 26: 124–129 Italy
10. UK wide survey on the Prevention of Post-ERCP Pancreatitis., Hanna, M.S. et al, Frontline Gastroenterology, 2014, 5: 103–110 UK
11. Increased Risk and Severity of ERCP-related complications associated with asymptomatic common bile duct stones., Saito, H. Kakuma, T., Kadono, Y., Urata, A., Kamakawa, K., Imamura, H., Tada, S., Endosc International, 2017, 5: E809–E817 Japan
12. Laparoscopic common bile duct exploration: A safe and definitive treatment for elderly patients., Zheng, C., Huang, Y., Xie, D., Peng, Y., Wang., Xiaozhong, Surg Endosc, 2017, 31: 2541–2547 China
13. Optimizing Choledocholithiasis Management., Poulouse, BK, et al, Arch Surg, 2007, 142: 43–48
14. Risk Factor of bleeding after Endoscopic Sphincterotomy in Average Risk Patients, Soo Bae, Sang et al., Surg Endosc, 2019, 33: 3334–3340 South Korea.

Laparoscopic Cholecystectomy: Introduction, Uptake, Maturity, and Impact on Surgical Practice—Personal Reflections from the Shop Floor

Alfred Cuschieri

Abstract

The essence of this new surgical approach is the reduction of the trauma of access; hence the appropriate name is *Minimal Access Surgery (MAS)*. Laparoscopic cholecystectomy has changed surgical practice across all the surgical disciplines and even changed current open surgical practice by earlier ambulation and reduction of hospital stay. The likely way ahead in specialist care of patients might well follow a new paradigm in the quest for improved patient outcome and further reduction of the traumatic insult to the patient by a new team approach of *MAT* (Minimal Access Therapy).

Keywords

Minimal Access Surgery · Laparoscopic surgery guidelines · Surgical controversies

Introduction

This chapter is based on personal experience as Chairman of the Department of Surgery, Molecular Oncology and Technology at the University of Dundee Scotland between 1st June 1976 and 30th September 2003, when I was fortunate enough to be offered a Chair of Surgery and Technology by the Italian Government until my return to Scotland as the Chief Scientific Advisor to the newly established *Institute for Medical Science and Technology* (IMSaT). When in Liverpool as lecturer and senior lecturer in the early 1970s, I developed a strong research interest in laparoscopy with its special application to oncology (lymphomas), the management of which at that time involved a staging laparotomy to exclude infradiaphragmatic disease. I was fortunate enough to be noticed by Professor David Weatherall, a prominent UK hematologist at the Royal Infirmary in Liverpool who subsequently was recruited as Professor of Medicine at the University of Oxford and duly knighted for his services to academic and clinical hematology. He encouraged me to undertake an initial laparoscopy trial and note findings before proceeding to the staging laparotomy and splenectomy, standard practice at the time. The correlation of the findings between laparoscopic staging and staging laparotomy was close. But what turned out to be my good fortune was a publication in the *British Journal of Surgery* of a paper entitled "Laparoscopy for the jaundice patient." This caught the attention of Dr George Berci, who personally invited me to Cedars Sinai Hospital in Los Angeles, where I gave two lectures, chaired by the late Dr Leon Morgenstern, Chairman of the Department of Surgery at Cedars, who was the most outstanding, cultured, and gifted human being I have ever encountered. As for Dr Berci, we became and remained close friends ever since.

In view of the complexity of the topic with so many issues and controversies, some of which persist to this day, the account is laid out in the following sections.

The original version of this chapter was revised. The correction to this chapter can be found at https://doi.org/10.1007/978-3-030-76845-4_20

Nomenclature and Origin of Laparoscopic Surgery/Cholecystectomy

Worldwide the new surgical approach is known and in well-established usage as *Minimally Invasive Surgery (MIS)*; but this is wrong as "to invade" is absolute. It is like saying "Hitler minimally invaded Poland and started world war II." Any breach of the skin by a needle, bee sting, whatever, can prove fatal in individuals with the innate genotypic susceptibility. The essence of the new surgical approach is the reduction of the trauma of access; hence the appropriate name is *Minimal Access Surgery (MAS)*. This is preferable to endoscopic surgery as this does not describe the essential features of the approach (Fig. 17.1).

In the controversy of who did the first laparoscopic cholecystectomy (LC), one needs to remind the readers that laparoscopic surgery as we know and practice it safely with dedicated technology with insufflation to safeguard the hemodynamic cardiovascular state during long periods of positive pressure ventilation, safe entry into the peritoneal cavity, and incredible imaging technology based on OLED colored monitors with 4 and 8 K resolution, including progressive 3D, has only come on the scene during the last 40 years. Hence the truth is that the advent of MAS is as much owed to technological advances in physics and optical engineering as it is to the early European pioneers, if not more. MAS LC followed the same maturation process (Fig. 17.2) as all other disruptive technologies, which change how humans live, communicate, and work. The term "disruptive technologies" was first described by Clayton M. Christensen of the Harvard Business School in his 1997 book, *The Innovator's Dilemma*.

The maturation of disruptive technologies progresses slowly along a complicated process initiated by a *Technology Trigger* (based on research and development (R&D) followed by an initial *peak of inflated expectations, then a trough of disillusionment (as limitations and problems are experienced), succeeded by a realistic upward slope of enlightenment as improved second generation products come on stream and lead to a high growth adoption of potential users of matured third generation products*. The technology underpinning MAS laparoscopic surgery followed the same maturation time frame of 25–30 years, but regrettably, was initially (for several years) a peripheral development as the main teaching hospitals and tertiary referral centers were, with a few exceptions, hesitant in their support for the new surgical approach.

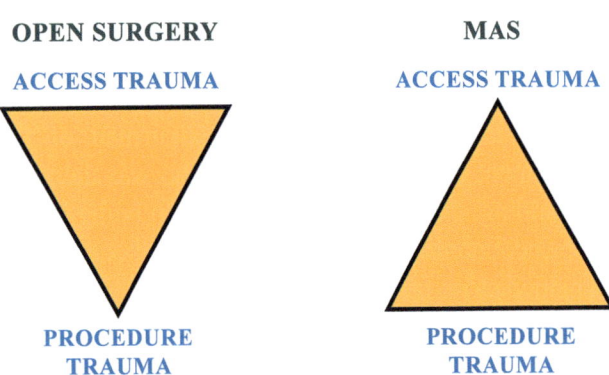

Fig. 17.1 Basic concept of MAS to reduce the trauma of access. Downside of MAS kinematic restriction to 4 degrees of freedom

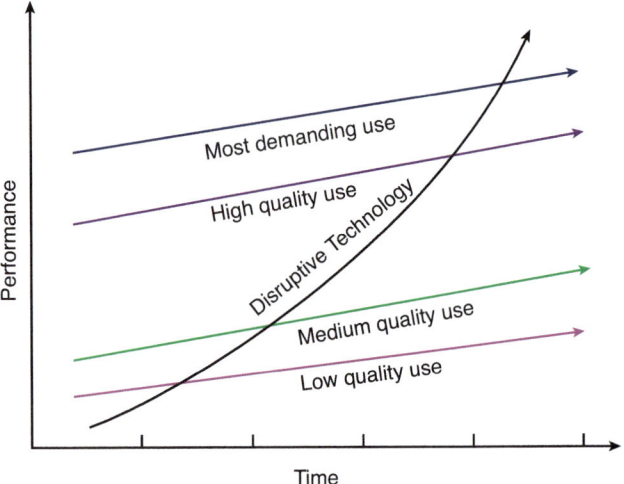

Fig. 17.2 08758458 Christensen Clayton M. (1997). *The Innovator's Dilemma*, Harvard Business School Press. ISBN 51

General Considerations

LC is a very common operation with an optimal clinical outcome in the vast majority of patients. In the United States alone, 500,000 LC operations are performed annually with an overall morbidity lower than 1.5%, and negligible mortality, averaging 0.1% [1]. However, the outcome is influenced by age, ASA status, and specific comorbid disorders exemplified by cirrhosis. The outcome of LC in patients with liver cirrhosis and symptomatic cholelithiasis not exceeding Child-Pugh A and B is well reported in the literature. These patients tend to be older than noncirrhotic patients undergoing LC for symptomatic cholelithiasis. They have a high conversion rate (averaging 16%), longer duration of hospital stay due to a postoperative unstable hemodynamic state, which may require high dependency or intensive care. In addition, they require a significantly longer postoperative hospital stay and incur major morbidity but with a low/acceptable mortality. Hence cirrhotic patients do not exceed Child-Pugh A and B stage, and they can be treated by LC for symptomatic gallstone disease [2, 3].

Increased risk in the elderly undergoing LC A recent study on postoperative risk of LC in the elderly was compared to younger patients by a systematic literature search of PubMed, EMBASE, and the Cochrane Library databases. This meta-analysis undertaken in accordance with the Cochrane Library and PRISMA guidelines reported on overall morbidity (primary endpoint) and conversion to open surgery, bile leaks, postoperative mortality, and length of stay (as secondary endpoints). The meta-analysis was based on 99 studies totaling 326,517 patients. Increasing age was significantly associated with increased overall morbidity (OR 2.37, CI 95% 2.00–2.78), major complication (OR 1.79, CI 95% 1.45–2.20), risk of conversion to open cholecystectomy (OR 2.17, CI 95% 1.84–2.55), risk of bile leaks (OR 1.50, CI 95% 1.07–2.10), risk of postoperative deaths (OR 7.20, CI 95% 4.41–11.73) in addition to increased length of stay (MD 2.21 days, CI 95% 1.24–3.18) [4].

Need for antibiotic prophylaxis (AP) Although various previous systematic reviews concluded that AP is not warranted in low-risk LC, many of these studies were underpowered with a relatively small sample size. Hence this view was never accepted by many surgeons who were proved right by the results of a recent prospective randomized controlled clinical trial (RCT). In this study, patients scheduled for elective LC were randomly assigned to two arms: those receiving AP and those who did not. The primary endpoint was the occurrence of postoperative infections, with secondary endpoints being postoperative hospital stay and medical costs. The study assigned 518 patients to receive AP and 519 who did not. Surgical site, distant and overall infections were significantly lower in the AP group compared to the no AP cohort (0.8 vs. 3.7%, $p = 0.001$, OR: 0.205 (95% CI: 0.069–0.606); 0.4 vs. 3.1%, $p = 0.0004$, OR: 0.122 (95% CI: 0.028–0.533); 1.2 vs. 6.7%; $p < 0.0001$, OR: 0.162 (95% CI: 0.068–0.389), respectively). The postoperative hospital stay was significantly shorter in the AP group (mean, SD: 3.69 ± 1.56 vs. 4.07 ± 3.00; $p = 0.01$) as were the postoperative medical costs in the AP group (mean, SD: $766 ± 341 vs. 832 ± 670; $p = 0.047$). Multivariable analysis confirmed as independent risk factors for postoperative infectious complications: no AP ($p < 0.0001$) and age 65 or older ($p = 0.006$). Hence AP is recommended in elective LC as it reduces postoperative infectious complications and medical costs [5].

Conversion to open surgery The importance of this aspect of good judgment is insufficiently stressed in the published literature. Conversion is best considered in two categories: *elective* and *enforced*. Elective conversion is defined as lack of material progress in the conduct of an operation most commonly because of adhesions from previous surgery or fibrosis in the porta hepatis/Calot's triangle region. There have been no studies that confirm the ideal duration of this period of trial dissection, but the consensus view is that it should not exceed 20 min of-non-productive attempts at safe exposure of the extrahepatic biliary tract. In contrast enforced conversion is required for a serious intraoperative iatrogenic injury or life-threatening hemorrhage.

One meta-analysis evaluated preoperative risk factors for conversion of LC to open cholecystectomy in all clinical studies published from 1990 to 2012 searched in the Med-line, Embase, Science Citation Index, and PubMed databases. Random and fixed-effect models were used to aggregate the study endpoints and assess heterogeneity. Eleven non-randomized clinical trials involving 14,645 patients (940 in the conversion (LOC) group and 13,705 in the LC group) were included in the meta-analysis. From the pooled analyses, age >65 years (OR = 1.83, 95% CI (1.31, 2.45), $p < 0.0001$), male gender (OR = 2.23, 95% CI (1.59, 3.12), $p < 0.00001$), diabetes mellitus (OR = 1.89, 95% CI (1.30, 2.75), $p = 0.0009$), acute cholecystitis (OR = 3.37, 95% CI (1.83, 6.20), $p < 0.0001$), thickened gallbladder wall (OR = 6.04, 95% CI (4.11, 8.88), $p < 0.00001$), and previous upper abdominal surgery (OR = 4.43, 95% CI (2.17, 9.04), $p < 0.00001$) were independent predictive risk factors for conversion. Previous lower abdominal surgery, preoperative endoscopic retrograde cholangiopancreatography (ERCP), and the gallstone pancreatitis were not significantly associated with conversion (all $p > 0.05$) [6]. Similar findings were reported by other studies including [7].

A large single center study reviewed the rate and causes of conversion from laparoscopic to open cholecystectomy (OC). It included all LCs for symptomatic gallstone disease undertaken from May 1999 to June 2010. The exclusion criteria were malignancy and/or existence of gallbladder polyps detected pathologically. Of 5382 patients in whom LC was attempted, 5164 were included in this study. The overall rate of conversion to OC was 3.16% (163 patients) consisting of 84 male and 79 female patients; mean age of 52.04 years (range, 26–85) with a female-to-male sex incidence of 5.6% and 2.2%, respectively ($p < 0.001$). The most common conversion rate was observed in males and in patients of both sexes with severe adhesions and fibrosis of Calot's triangle. The overall postoperative morbidity rate was 16.3% in patients who were converted to open surgery [8].

Bile duct leaks in the absence of major bile duct injury The management of bile leaks following LC in a minimally invasive management protocol. Reported in a series of 24 patients with a bile leak following consecutively between two periods: (i) 10 patients between 1993 and 2003 were managed on a case-by-case basis and (ii) 14 between 1998 and 2003 were managed according to a minimally invasive protocol utilizing ERC/biliary stenting and re-laparoscopy if indicated. Bile leaks presented as bile in a drain left in situ post LC (8/10 vs. 10/14) or biliary peritonitis (2/10 vs. 4/14). Prior to 1998, neither ERC nor laparoscopy was in routine use locally. During this period, 4/10 patients recovered with conservative management and 6/10 (60%) underwent laparotomy. There was one postoperative death and median hospital stay post LC was 10 days (range, 5–30 days). In the protocol era, ERC ± stenting was performed in 11/14 ($p = 0.01$ vs. pre-protocol) with the main indication being a persistent bile leak. Re-laparoscopy was necessary in 5/14 ($p = 0.05$ vs. pre-protocol). No laparotomies were performed ($p < 0.01$ vs. pre-protocol) and there were no postoperative deaths. Median hospital stay was 11 days (range, 5–55 days). The results of this study confirmed the introduction of a minimally invasive protocol utilizing ERC and re-laparoscopy offers an effective modern algorithm for the management of bile leaks after LC [9].

ERCP with placement of a biliary stent or nasobiliary (NB) drain is the procedure of choice for treatment of post-cholecystectomy bile duct leaks. The study compared the effect of NB vs. internal biliary stenting on rates of leak closure, time elapsed until drain or stent removal, length of hospital stay, and number of endoscopic procedures required. The study involved 20 patients who underwent LC complicated by Luschka or cystic duct leaks, 10 of whom were treated with NB drains connected to low intermittent suction and repeat NB cholangiograms performed until leak closure. Another 10 patients were treated with insertion of internal biliary stents. Biliary sphincterotomies were performed for stone extraction or a presumed papillary stenosis. Large bilomas were drained percutaneously prior to stenting.

In all 20 patients, a cholangiogram and successful placement of an NB drain or internal stent was achieved. Four patients (20%) were found to have ductal stones, which were extracted following a sphincterotomy. Sixteen patients required percutaneous drainage of large bilomas prior to biliary instrumentation. Ten biliary leaks (15 from cystic duct leaks and 5 ducts of Luschka) were reviewed. Closure of the leak was documented within 2–11 days (mean 4.7 ± 0.9 days) in patients receiving an NB drain. The drains were removed non-endoscopically following leak closure. The internal stent group required stenting for 14–53 days (mean 29.1 ± 4.4 days). The stent was then removed endoscopically after documented closure of leaks. Bile leaks following LC closed rapidly after NB drainage and did not require repeat endoscopy for removal of the NB drain, resulting in fewer ERCPs required for their treatment. Internal biliary stents were in place longer owing to the nature of this intermittent endoscopic approach but an accurate comparison of time to leak closure could not be determined. Leak closure resulted once the bile flow was reestablished. However, removal of NB drains was performed earlier than removal of the biliary stents. The number of ERCPs required per patient was 1.0 ± 0 in the NB group and 2.2 ± 0.1 (range, 2–3) in the internal stent group. The length of hospitalization was 8.7 ± 3.3 days for the NB group and 7.5 ± 2.3 days for the internal stent group. Biliary stent placement resulted in an insignificant decrease in hospitalization at the expense of requiring twice as many endoscopic procedures. This study suggests that NB drainage may be advantageous in patients requiring a prolonged hospital admission or in patients in whom repeat endoscopy is undesirable. Internal biliary stenting appears preferable when early discharge is anticipated or when expertise in placement and management of NB drains is not available or lacking [10].

Early recognition of complications after LC Enables prompt intervention and may lead to an improved patient outcome. Imaging studies are necessary to exclude biloma, hematoma, and abscess formation. However, a small amount of fluid in the gallbladder fossa is commonly seen postoperatively on ultrasonography (US). Dilatation of intrahepatic ducts is always significant and indicative of obstruction either from retained stones or iatrogenic bile duct injury. The use of hemostatic agents placed in the gallbladder bed, for example, oxidized regenerated cellulose is inadvisable as when imaged during postoperative period, it can be mistaken for a hematoma, abscess [11, 12], or less commonly, tumor [13, 14].

Initial Nosocomial Surgical Epidemic

The first large reported retrospective series of LC was based on data from seven European centers involving 20 surgeons who undertook 1236 LCs. The operation was completed in 1191 patients. Conversion to open cholecystectomy was necessary in 45 patients (3.6%) either because of technical difficulty ($n = 33$), the onset of complications ($n = 11$), or stapler disposable instrument failure ($n = 1$). There were no deaths reported, and the total postoperative complication rate was 20 of 1203 (1.6%), with nine being serious complications requiring laparotomy. The total incidence of bile duct damage was 4 of 1203 (*0.003*). The median hospital stay was 3 days (range, 1–27 days) and the median time to return to full activity after discharge was 11 days (range, 7–42 days) [15]. The article concluded that LC was safe but failed to realize that we had initiated a maelstrom which lasted several years. In retrospect the reason for this initial nosocomial surgical epidemic were several. In the first instance, with few exceptions of a few European and North American centers, most of the mainstream teaching hospitals and tertiary referral centers refused to back the new MAS approach. Consequently, LC uptake was initially a peripheral uncontrolled development since it predated Institutional Review Boards (IRBs) and Credentialing with granting of privileges to attending surgeons; and their equivalent in other countries. This being the case, in most instances when adopting new technologies and surgical approaches, most physicians tend to be guided by their sense of professionalism and duty of care, in avoiding any harm to the patients they treat and are wary of potential lawsuits. Additionally, hospitals share the medicolegal risks by establishing and confirming the qualifications of licensed attending physicians and by authorizing them for specific patient care services (privileging).

None of the above checks existed anywhere during the period 1988–1993. One prominent highly respected surgical academic, who served on the editorial board of the *New England Journal of Medicine*, called it "the greatest irresponsible free for all in the history of surgery." The situation was compounded by two additional contributing cofactors: one involving the few surgeons on both sides of the Atlantic, who were involved as pioneers in the training of surgeons in the MAS laparoscopic approach to ensure competence in the execution of LC and other MAS operations, as fully competent surgeons who in turn trained others on a scheme referred as "training the trainers." The unwitting error in the training process enacted by these trainers (myself included) was the introduction and use of edited videos of LC and other operations which proved counterproductive. These edited videos by removing technical errors imparted the wrong message that safe execution LC and other laparoscopic procedures was easy for any surgeon fully trained in conventional open surgery. This practice was an error of judgment, as it failed to recognize the importance of training and skills acquisition of technical errors, especially how to avoid them or the remedial actions needed.

The initial nosocomial epidemic was characterized by two dramatic consequences: major bile duct injuries and vascular injuries with catastrophic hemorrhage.

Major bile duct injuries MBDI Overall, MBDI enacted during LC increased fivefold worldwide, all being serious and, in a small subset, life threatening. The latter are patients who sustained combined vascular-MBDI, as in essence, they developed acute or chronic liver failure from secondary biliary cirrhosis with end-stage liver disease requiring liver transplant (LT) for survival. Furthermore, a substantial cohort, despite obtaining improved liver function with subsidence of jaundice and itching improved by reconstructive hepaticojejunostomy, remains subject to episodes of recurrent cholangitis for the rest of their lives.

Clinically patients who sustain MBDI are severely ill and jaundiced with intermittent fever. They complain of abdominal pain requiring analgesic medication and exhibit abdominal tenderness with rebound from biliary peritonitis. One review of their management concluded that they are best avoided by careful dissection of the key structures and correct interpretation of the anatomy. This review stresses the importance of routine, as opposed to selective, intraoperative cholangiography (IOC) which is associated with a lower incidence of MBDI and their early recognition. It also stresses the importance of early detection and repair in ensuring an improved patient outcome. However, there is controversy on the optimal time for surgical reconstruction. The authors of this review indicate that the minimum standard of care after the recognition of MBDI consists of immediate referral to a surgeon or experienced unit with the resources to manage and repair these complex injuries [16].

A small subset of patients with combined vascular and MBD requires liver transplantation (LT) for survival. Several large series have been reported from both sides of the Atlantic [17–20].

There has been only one prospective case registration based on a national database with participation by all Departments of Surgery performing LC in Denmark undertaken since the first operation *in* January 1991. During this period, 57 of 7654 patients sustained bile duct injury (0.74%; 95% CI, 0.55–0.94%), including nine injuries occurring after conversion. The annual incidence during the entire study period did not change. Thirty-nine percent of the laparoscopic bile duct injuries (BDI) were incisions, 39% were transections, and 12% were clip injuries or strictures. One patient, who sustained transection during open reoperation for bleeding during the converted operation, died. Acute cholecystitis was the indication for LC in 968 patients, with 1.3% sustaining laparoscopic BDI (95% CI 0.62–2.08%), while the incidence in patients with other indications for LC was lower at 0.62% (95% CI 0.44–0.82%) ($p > 0.05$). Preoperative knowledge of bile duct anatomy was available in 26% of patients undergoing LC but this did not reduce the risk of BDI. The frequency of BDI in patients who had intraoperative cholangiography was not significantly different from those who did not.

Conclusions The main conclusion from this national registry study is that the incidence of BDI in LC is higher than previously generally anticipated and did not decrease from 1991 through 1994 [21].

Optimal time for reconstruction of MBDI Except for patients with combined vascular and MBDI requiring urgent LT for acute liver failure, there has been an ongoing controversy regarding the optimal timing of surgical reconstruction after MBDI. To a large extent, this has been resolved by systematic review designed to establish the optimal time for remedial surgery usually in a tertiary referral center. The search used PubMed, Embase, and Cochrane databases for publications between 1990 and 2018 reporting on the timing of hepaticojejunostomy for MBDI (PROSPERO registration CRD42018106611). The main outcome measures for the systemic review were: postoperative morbidity, postoperative mortality, and anastomotic stricture. Data for comparable time intervals were pooled using a random-effects model. In addition, data for all included studies were pooled using a generalized linear model. Twenty-one studies were included, representing 2484 patients. The study looked at the outcome following different time intervals: (i) 8 with time intervals of less than 14 days (*early*), (ii) 14 days–6 weeks (*intermediate*), and (iii) > than 6 weeks (*delayed*). Meta-analysis revealed a higher risk of postoperative morbidity in the intermediate interval; *early* vs. *intermediate*: risk ratio (RR) 0·73, 95% CI 0·54–0·98; *intermediate* vs. *delayed*: RR 1·50, 1·16–1·93. Stricture rate was lowest in the delayed interval group; *intermediate* vs. *delayed*: RR 1·53, 1·07–2·20. Postoperative mortality did not differ between time intervals. Additional analysis demonstrated increased odds of postoperative morbidity for reconstruction between 2 and 6 weeks, and decreased odds of anastomotic stricture for delayed reconstruction.

The important conclusion of this study is that surgical reconstruction of MDBI between 2 and 6 weeks should be avoided as this was associated with higher risk of postoperative morbidity and hepaticojejunostomy stricture [22].

Major vascular injuries (MVI) sustained during LC These injuries are rare nowadays; most being reported during the first decade following introduction of LC. They can occur during the creation of the positive pressure capnoperitoneum usually when undertaken with the closed technique using a Veress needle, during the insertion of ports especially the first (for the optic), during the conduction of the LC, and even after conversion to open surgery (OC) or even with the open Hasson technique [23]. Although no vessel is immune, the common MVI injuries which are immediately life threatening from exsanguination involve the infradiaphragmatic aorta, the portal vein, and the inferior vena cava.

Vascular injuries sustained during creation of positive pressure capnoperitoneum One meta-analysis evaluated the reported incidence of both vascular and visceral injuries encountered with closed vs. open capnoperitoneum induction. It revealed 336 major vascular injuries in 760,890 closed laparoscopies, a mean rate of 0.044%, 1 injury per 2272 cases, compared with no injuries in 22,465 open laparoscopies ($p = 0.003$). Visceral injuries were more frequent, 515 injuries in 760,890 closed laparoscopies (mean rate = 0.07) vs. 1 injury in 22,465 open laparoscopies (mean rate = 0.05; $p = 0.18$). Hence, this report shows that open laparoscopy eliminates the risk of major vascular injury and reduces the rate of major visceral injuries. Open laparoscopy using the Hasson cannula should be the preferred method of peritoneal access [24].

Vascular injuries during conduct of LC Major vascular injury most commonly occurs during the laparoscopic entry phase. It is commoner with closed entry (Veress needle) and in recent years has been reported a range of specialties including in urologic procedures. One such study involved a series of 5347 patients who underwent laparoscopic urologic operation between 1996 and 2011 in patients in whom entry was carried out by either the closed Veress needle technique or the modified open Hasson technique. The closed technique was used in the first 474 operations, and in a much larger subsequent cohort of 4873 patients, the creation of the capnoperitoneum was by the open Hasson technique. Three patients sustained major vascular injury all undergoing nephrectomy, with all being sustained in the initial closed capnoperitoneum group during the setup phase and insertion of the first trocar. The injuries involved the abdominal aorta in two patients and the external iliac vein in a third patient. It is difficult to draw any robust conclusion from this study [25].

Techniques of Laparoscopic Cholecystectomy

Attempts have been made to reduce the traumatic insult to the patient and to improve cosmesis and reduce scarring. Some of these have been ill advised as they increase the level of difficulty of execution. These include single port laparoscopic surgery (SILS) also referred to as reduced port surgery [26, 27] and many others. Another publication is important because it quantitated the extra costs incurred by SILS-LC vs. conventional 4 port LC [28].

The publication aimed to calculate the cost of the operating time to demonstrate that SILS-LC is significantly more expensive than conventional LC. It identified studies comparing use of SILS LC vs. conventional LC during the period 2008–2016 together with another search to calculate the costs during the same time interval. A meta-analysis was then performed of the items selected in the first review relating to costs of surgery and surgical time and calculated the differences based on the cost/time variable using the data from the second review. Twenty-seven articles were selected from the first review: 26 for operating time (3138 patients) and three for the cost of surgery (831 patients), together with three articles from the second review. Both SILS-LC and conventional 4 port LC have similar operating costs. However, as SILS-LC takes longer (17 min) to perform ($p < 0.00001$), this difference represents an opportunity cost of 755.97 € (cost/time unit factor of 44.73 €/min).

The quest toward reduction of the access trauma over the past five decades is illustrated in Fig. 17.3.

In the author's opinion, the best approach which does not affect the degree of difficulty in carrying out not only LC but other more complex MAS laparoscopic operations which require intracorporeal suturing without leaving discernible external scarring or additional operating costs is needlescopic surgery [29].

Conventional vs. retrograde (fundus first) LC Fundus first LC (FF-LC) has gained popularity since its first introduction in 1995 in view of its advantages and increased safety over conventional LC based on initial trial dissection of the cystic artery and duct within the triangle of Calot, especially in the presence of severe acute cholecystitis,

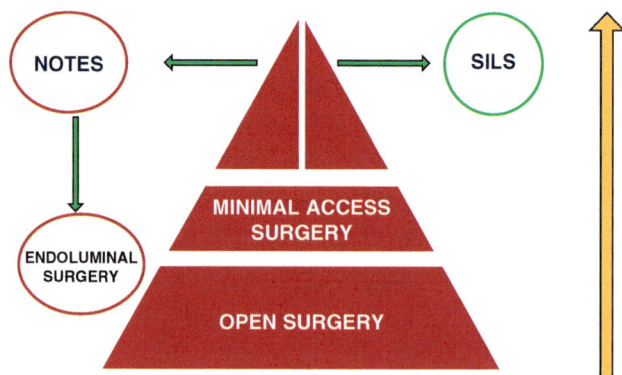

Fig. 17.3 Schematic illustration of the two approaches in the quest (vertical arrow) toward reduction of access trauma and external scarring. SILS has become increasingly underutilized in the last 5 years, whereas NOTES has been the forerunner of endoluminal intramural surgery, exemplified by POEM

Mirizzi syndrome, and anomalous anatomy of the extrahepatic biliary tract [30–36].

FF-LC is certainly a cost-effective way to simplify execution of LC and appears to facilitate patient rehabilitation and has become very popular in Scandinavian countries since the reported large retrospective series by Cengiz et al. in 2019. Between 2004 and 2014, 29 surgeons performed 1425 LC with FF and 320 with the conventional technique. During the first year 56% used the FF technique as distinct from 98% during remaining years. The FF-LC cohort contained more female patients, urgent operations, day care operations, and averaged a shorter operation time and an overall morbidity in 63 (3.6%): 0.6% bleeding, 1.9% infections, and 0.7% bile leakages: from cystic 4/112 when sealed with ultrasonic shears and in 4/1633 (0.2%) with clips (p 0.008). One common bile duct lesion occurred in 1/1425 (0.07%) and in 3/320 (0.9%) with the conventional LC (p 0.003). In a multivariate regression, the conventional LC technique was a risk factor for bile duct injury with an odds ratio of 20.8 (95% CI 1.6–259.2) [37].

Patients with Symptomatic Gallstones and Ductal Calculi

The management of these patients remains clouded in controversy, entrenched views without the necessary evidence in the current era of evidence based as opposed to eminence-based medical practice to which all clinicians should subscribe to. The issue is based on the established fact that many common bile duct stones remain clinically "silent" without any symptoms or apparent harm to the individuals concerned. Worldwide, the vast majority of surgeons *estimated at 90% plus* do not perform any intraoperative visualization of the biliary tract in patients undergoing LC for symptomatic gallstones on the basis of available evidence including results of RCTs even if statistically underpowered [38].

A smaller subset of surgeons adopted a selective approach to intraoperative cholangiography (IOC) most commonly by iodinated contrast media (Fig. 17.4) and more recently by indocyanine green (ICG) cholangiography [39–41].

The options for the treatment of patients with common bile duct stones (CBD) stones are: (i) preoperative ERCP for duct extraction followed by LC, (ii) single-stage LC and laparoscopic-endoscopic rendezvous ERCP extraction, and (iii) intraoperative ductal stone clearance by either direct supraduodenal CBD exploration or by the trans-cystic basket trawling technique if the stones are small (>6 mm).

A Cochrane Database Systematic Review compared the benefits and morbidity of endoscopic sphincterotomy, and stone removal followed by LC with the single-stage rendezvous technique in patients with symptomatic cholelithiasis harboring CBD stones. This review included five RCTs with 517 participants (257 underwent a laparoscopic-endoscopic rendezvous technique (LRVT) vs. 260

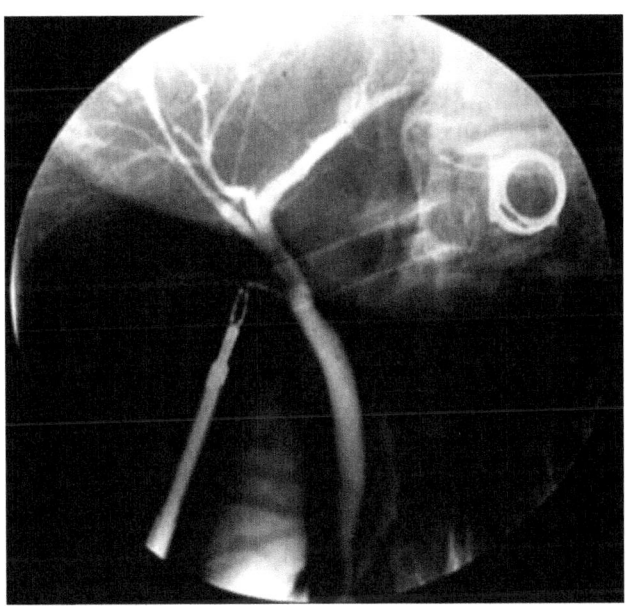

Fig. 17.4 Contrast IOC with slow injection to avoid overfilling of the biliary tree during radiologic imaging by image intensifier. The problem with the selective approach with slow trans cystic duct injection of contrast with concomitant image intensifier imaging (essential to avoid overfilling which obscures small calculi) is that cannulation and securing a ureteric catheter into the cystic duct is virtually impossible or adds considerably to the operative time if not performed routinely. This is the Achilles heel of the selective approach

treated by the standard two-stage sequential approach). Overall, the five trials were judged at high risk of bias. Only one patient in the LRVT group died. The overall morbidity (surgical and general) was lower in the LRVT cohort (RR 0.59, 95% CI 0.29–1.20; participants = 434, trials = 4; $I^2 = 28\%$); but appeared slightly more robust when a fixed-effect model was used (RR 0.56, 95% CI 0.32–0.99). There was no difference between the two approaches on primary clearance of CBD stones. The effects of either approach on incidence of postoperative pancreatitis are not clear. Hospital stay in the two-stage sequential approach exceeded LRVT by 3 days but the LRVT procedure incurred a longer, but insignificant, operating time [42].

An RCT compared two management options. Group A ($n = 150$) received preoperative endoscopic retrograde cholangiography (ERC) with ES followed by LC during the same hospital admission, and group B ($n = 150$) received single-stage laparoscopic management: There were no significant differences between the two groups in the clinical demographic details and the pretreatment biochemical findings. In group A, 14 of 150 patients received single-stage treatment; in group B, 17 of 150 were managed by the two-stage approach (protocol violation = 31/300, 10%). In group A patients managed in accordance with randomization, ERC was successful in 129/136 (95%) and preoperative ES was successful in stone clearance in 82/98 (84%). As two patients had malignancies and one refused surgery, 133 patients underwent surgery. In this group, 116 patients had LC only and 17 had LC and attempted laparoscopic CBD exploration. There were eight conversions to open surgery (6%), 17 complications for both stages (12.8%), and two postoperative deaths (1.5%). For patients in group B who were managed in accordance with randomization, IOC was successful in 132/133 (99%). Twenty-one (16%) had normal findings, ductal calculi were found in 109, and other pathology was noted in two (periampullary cancer, severe pancreatitis). These two patients and another who had gross adhesion in the triangle of Calot were converted at the start of the procedure. Transcystic ductal stone clearance was successful in 45 of 56 patients (80%), and laparoscopic direct common duct (CBD) exploration was successful in 47 of 55 patients (85%). This group includes 53 patients who underwent primary direct exploration and two failed attempts at transcystic extraction. The conversion rate was 13%. Postoperative complications were encountered in 21 patients (15.8%), and one patient died of a major myocardial infarction (0.75%). The one postoperative death and the 11 biliary complications occurred in the laparoscopic supraduodenal CBD exploration subgroup. The conversion rate was higher in group B (17 vs 8; $p = 0.08$). Laparotomy in the postoperative period was required in three patients in group A and four patients in group B. The hospital stay in group B patients was 3 days less than patients who had two-stage management (median, 6.0, IQR = 4.25–12 vs median, 9.0, IQR = 5.5–14; $p < 0.05$) [43].

It is the author's practice to suture the choledochotomy after evacuation of stone by supraduodenal choledochotomy after the insertion of a special silicon cannula which is tied in place and connected to a closed bile drainage bag. A postoperative cholangiogram is performed the next day and if normal, the silicon cannula is closed and the patient is discharged 24 h later and returned for removal of the cannula as an outpatient 2 weeks later (Fig. 17.5).

Day Case/Ambulatory LC

One report from Japan evaluated the feasibility and safety of ambulatory LC with day case discharge or need for an overnight stay. The data from patients undergoing ambulatory LC were collected retrospectively and consecutively for patients requiring at least one overnight hospital stay over a two-year period. There were no hospital deaths or readmissions with serious morbidity after discharge. Fifty patients received day case LC and 19 had a required overnight stay. These patients were significantly older ($p < 0.02$). No significant differences were observed between the day case LC performed ($n = 41$) and failed ($n = 9$) and between the day case LC performed and requiring one-night stay LC ($n = 12$) groups. A

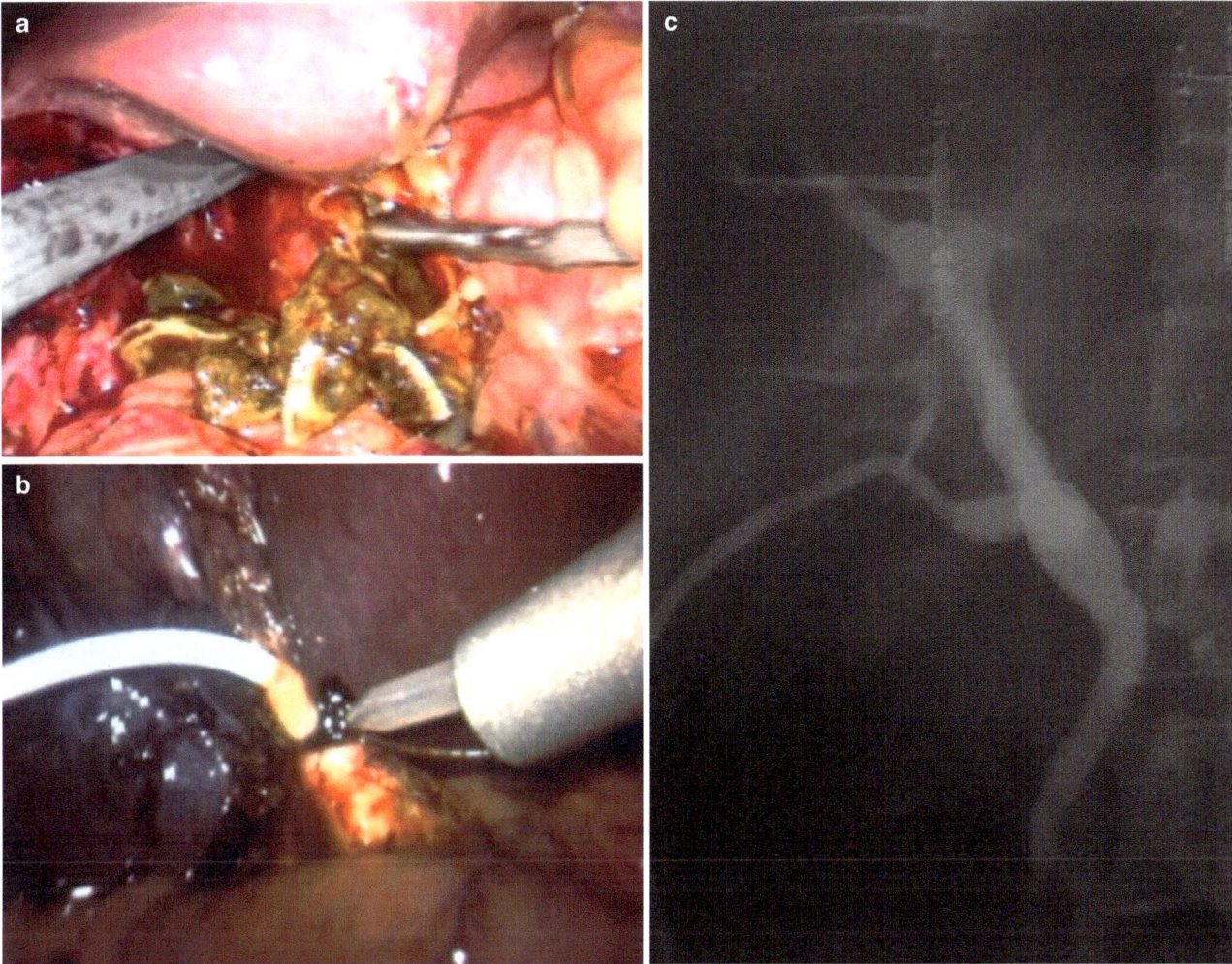

Fig. 17.5 (**a**) A supraduodenal CBD duct stone clearance, (**b**) 3 mm silicone cannula inserted into the CBD and tied in place to cystic duct stump, (**c**) postoperative cholangiogram confirming clearance

significant age difference was also observed between patients requiring one or more night's stay ($p < 0.05$). The important message from this study is that day case LC can be performed with a low rate of complications in elderly patients with some needing an overnight hospital stay, although many could be discharged the same day [43, 44].

It is important to stress that many RCTs conducted worldwide confirm the benefits, social and economic, of day case LC. Hence it is important to highlight the RCT reported from India by Kumar et al. [45]. This RCT recruited 65 patients with symptomatic gallstone who were randomized to either day case LC or routine elective operation. The assessment included quality of life, satisfaction, postoperative nausea, and vomiting and pain. Ninety-seven percent (31/32) of day case LC patients were successfully discharged with mean duration of 8.9 ± 4.54 h, compared to 3.33 ± 1.45 days (72.92 ± 34.8 h) in routine elective in hospital LC group. This RCT found no significant difference in morbidity, quality of life, satisfaction, postoperative nausea and vomiting, and pain between the two groups.

Bleeding Complications Associated with LC

Although the reported incidence of bleeding complications requiring transfusion after LC is rare, occurring in 0.1% in patients, serious major life-threatening vascular complications do occur [46]. Major bleeding during execution of LC is also a frequent indication for conversion [47]. The Finnish Register study [48] compared the bleeding complications, transfusion rates, and related costs between LC and open cholecystectomy (OC) in the period between 2002 and 2007 based on blood component use between 2002 and 2007 collected from existing computerized medical records (Finnish Red Cross Register) of ten Finnish hospital districts. In total, 22,117 cholecystectomies were performed during the study period, accounting for 43% all cholecystectomies (51,094) performed in Finland in 2002–2007. The study data sets comprised 17,175 LCs (78%) and 4942 (22%) OCs. In the OC much smaller cohort, 16% of patients received blood component transfusion compared to 1.6% of the patients in the LC group. Likewise, the proportions of patient with RBC (13% vs. 1.3%, $p < 0.001$), PLT (1.2% vs. 0.1%, $p < 0.001$), FFP (4.9% vs. 0.4%, $p < 0.001$), and Octaplas® (0.9% vs. 0.1%, $p < 0.001$) transfusions were all respectively higher in OC group compared to the LC group, as was the mean transfused dose of the FFP. There is thus no doubt that the laparoscopic MAS approach drastically reduces blood component transfusion.

Training and Simulation

This was initiated in Western countries with the establishment of Surgical Skills Units specifically for hands-on training in MAS laparoscopic surgery. The first such unit in Europe was established in October 1992 at Ninewells Hospital and Medical School in Dundee Scotland funded by industry and donations from Lord Wolfson, various Scottish Trusts; subsequently renamed as the Cuschieri Skills Center (CSC). It has been run since then by a medically qualified director, with a dedicated team of trained technicians and local surgeons. The CSC has served as a template for other such units in the UK and mainland European countries, with the emphasis that hands-on training accounts for 70% of the course content. Over the years, the CSC has progressed from use of synthetic models, trainer boxes containing animal tissue models to advanced virtual reality simulators for surgery including robotic-assisted surgery and flexible upper GI endoscopy and colonoscopy. But the promising and important development to the CSC has been the introduction of the use of the soft embalmed human corpses by a process developed by Prof Thiel in Graz [49, 50] and validated by the IMSaT Group of interface scientists in Dundee and others [50, 51]. The R&D over the years at IMSaT and the CSC has convinced me that it is by far and away the best way to train for both MAS laparoscopic surgery and open surgical operations than any advanced VR simulator both for anatomical teaching and for advanced procedure-related interventions. The human corpses are so life like in color and tissue elasticity that one BBC news commentary indicated that it was like "operating on the living dead." Perhaps I should add that I have been concerned with the use of fresh human corpses (including body parts) used in many countries including the UK since aside from the unbelievable stench which pervades the wet lab skills, I have concerns about potential health hazards to both trainee participants and tutors. In the UK, the Thiel embalming operated legally by means of a living will whereby any UK citizen, under the Anatomy Act, can donate his or her body immediately after death for soft embalming to UK Universities for research and medical training. The universities taking on this important commitment become the official holders of the corpses and must ultimately bury or cremate according to the wishes of the individual donors (Figs. 17.6 and 17.7).

Impact of LC on Surgical Practice across the Specialties

There is no question that humanity has benefitted with the onset of LC and the MAS laparoscopic approach. LC has changed surgical practice across all the surgical disciplines and even changed current open surgical practice by earlier ambulation and reduction of hospital stay. In transplant surgery, living-related donor nephrectomies have increased threefold in Western countries and the period of warm ischemia has reduced. The same increase has been reported in living-related split liver transplantation in Western countries, especially in children (Fig. 17.8).

Fig. 17.6 Comparison of formalin and (**a**) Thiel soft embalmed human knee joints (**b**)

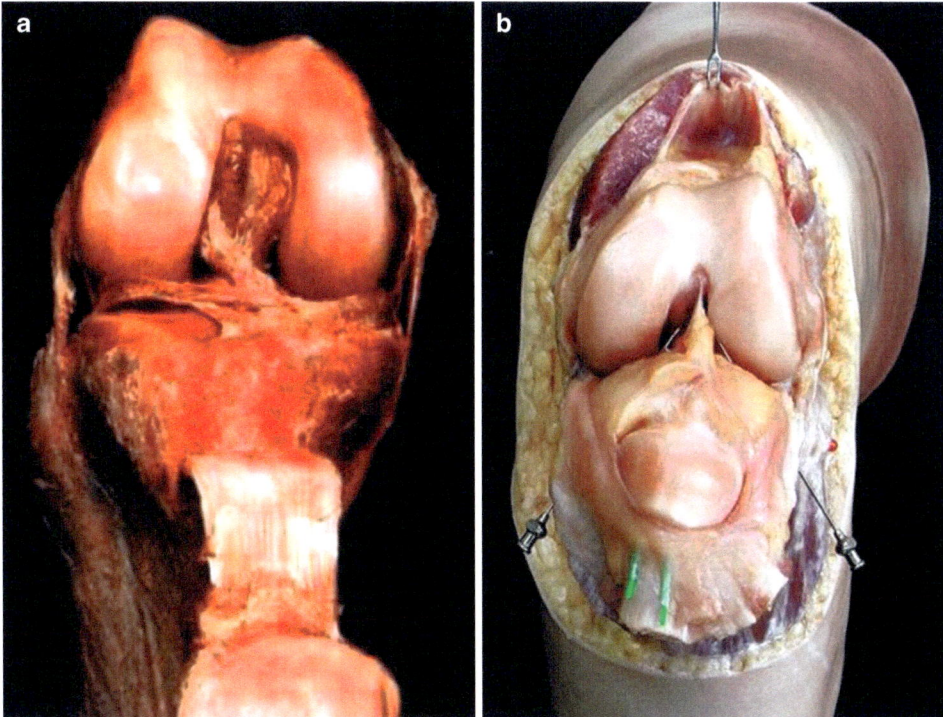

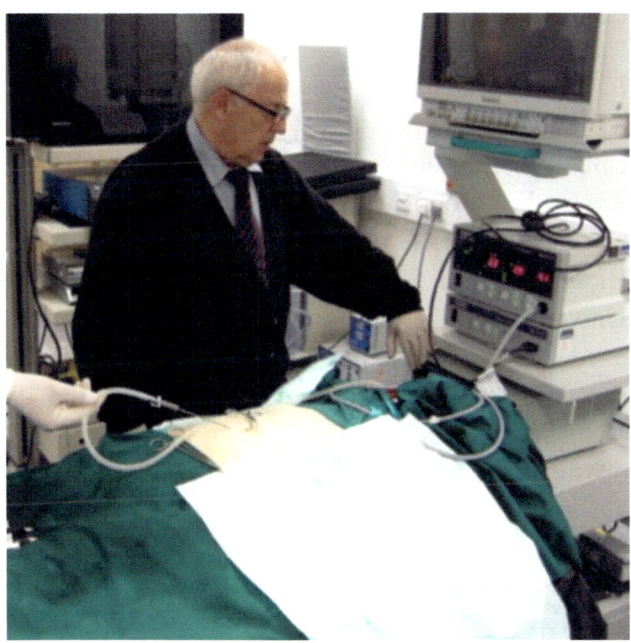

Fig. 17.7 Insufflation of peritoneal cavity in a Thiel soft embalmed human corpse

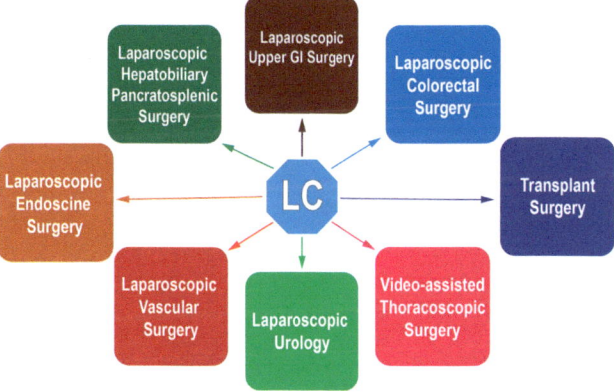

Fig. 17.8 Transformation of surgery by LC across the surgical disciplines

Like other disruptive developments, the underpinning technologies involved have now reached the fourth generation with HD CCD cameras and colored 4 and 8 K resolution organic light-emitting diodes (OLED) monitors which produce less heat, with excellent color rendition and wide viewing angle.

Even so, imaging will eventually change to *frontal gaze down imaging on top of the patient's chest* following 20 years of R&D by the author with two visual psychologists (Figs. 17.9 and 17.10).

The research underpinning frontal gaze down imaging demonstrate the optimal position of the image display influences both the efficiency (execution time) and the quality of the task/operation when:

(i) The image is placed at the level of the surgeon's hands—work plane.

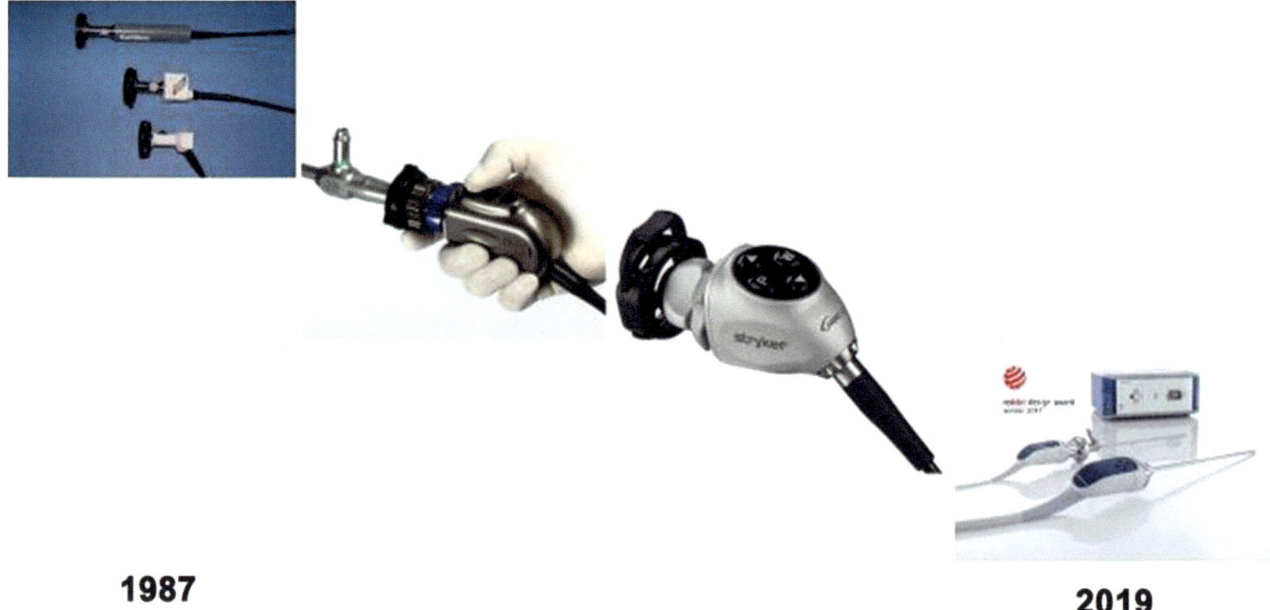

Fig. 17.9 Progress in endocameras to HD/optoelectronic telescopes

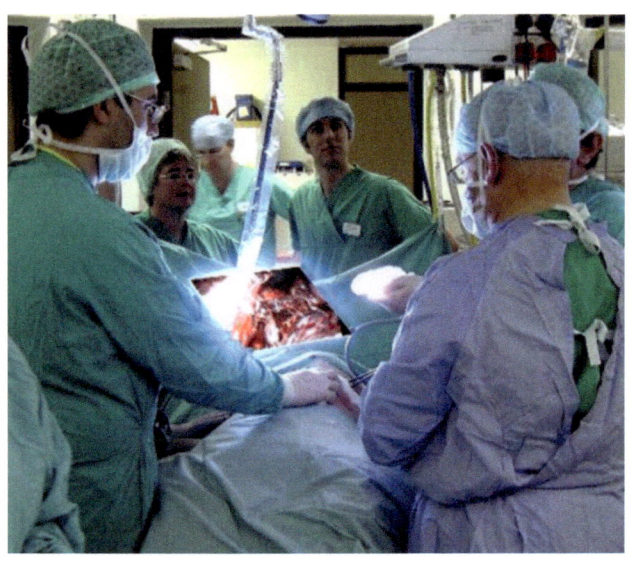

Fig. 17.10 Image projection onto a sterile specially textured screen enabling the surgeon (AC) to operate and manipulate in the same plane as his hands. The operation MAS laparoscopic R_2 gastrectomy for gastric cancer

(ii) The image is located directly in front and below the head of the operating surgeon, enabling "gaze-down frontal viewing."
(iii) The hands of the surgeon are in the same plane as the image.
(iv) The image is close to the actual operation site—reduces the cerebral mapping problem (Kennedy and Wade).

Advent of Robotically Assisted Laparoscopic Surgery

It was inevitable that the kinematic restriction of MAS laparoscopic surgery would lead to robotically assisted surgery and after initial work by the Karlsruhe group in Germany led by the late Gerhard Buess, DARPA then directed by Dr. Richard Satava donated a large grant to Stanford University for the development of robotic telepresence surgery, which ultimately led to the establishment of Intuitive Surgery that marketed the da Vinci Master Slave surgical manipulator, thereby opening a new chapter not of robotic surgery (as yet anyway) but as Robotic-assisted Laparoscopic Surgery.

What Next?

Although it is risky to make predictions, the likely way ahead in specialist care of patients might well follow a new paradigm in the quest for improved patient outcome and further reduction of the traumatic insult to the patient by a new team approach of *MAT* (Minimal Access Therapy). In this MAT approach, operations will be renamed interventions. MAT will encompass specialist physicians dedicated to the treatment of serious life-threatening disorders, hence collectively known as Disease Related Treatment Groups (DRTGs). Separate DRTGs will address CARDIAC, CANCER, INFECTIONS, and TRAUMA. Each DRTG will incorporate interventional radiologists largely operating high TESLA MRI systems, interventional flexible endoscopists, traumatologists, and minimal access surgical interventionalists. In practice, each DRTG will discuss and decide on the most appropriate treatment of individual patients based on stage of the disease, ASA status, and age.

References

1. Osborne DA, Alexander G, Boe B, Zervos EE. Laparoscopic cholecystectomy: past, present, and future. Surg Technol Int 2006; 15:81–5.
2. Eduardo B V da Silveira. Outcome of cirrhotic patients undergoing cholecystectomy: applying Bayesian analysis in gastroenterology. J Gastroenterol Hepatol. 2006;21(6):958–62. https://doi.org/10.1111/j.1440-1746.2006.04227. PMID: 16724978
3. TE Pavlidis, NG Symeonidis, K Psarras, C Skouras et al. Laparoscopic cholecystectomy in patients with cirrhosis of the liver and symptomatic cholelithiasis. JSLS. 2009;13(3):342–5. PMID: 19793474 PMCID: PMC3015965.
4. Sivesh K Kamarajah, Santhosh Karri, James R. Bundred et al. Perioperative outcomes after laparoscopic cholecystectomy in elderly patients: a systematic review and meta-analysis. Surg Endosc. 2020; 34(11): 4727–4740. https://doi.org/10.1007/s00464-020-07805-z.
5. Y Matsui, S Satoi, M Kaibori et al. Antibiotic prophylaxis in laparoscopic cholecystectomy: a randomized controlled trial PLoS One. 2014; 9(9): e106702. https://doi.org/10.1371/journal.pone.0106702. PMCID: PMC4156368.
6. TF Yang, L Guo, Q Wang. Evaluation of preoperative risk factor for converting laparoscopic to open cholecystectomy: a meta-analysis Hepatogastroenterology. 2014;61(132):958–65. PMID: 26158149.
7. N W Lee, J Collins, R Britt and L D Britt. Evaluation of preoperative risk factors for converting laparoscopic to open cholecystectomy Am Surg. 2012;78(8):831–3. PMID: 22856487.
8. V Genc, M Sulaimanov, G Cipe et al. What necessitates the conversion to open cholecystectomy? A retrospective analysis of 5164 consecutive laparoscopic operations. Clinics (Sao Paulo). 2011;66(3):417–420. https://doi.org/10.1590/S1807-59322011000300009. PMCID: PMC3072001 PMID: 21552665.
9. F Ahmad, R N Saunders, G M Lloyd et al. An algorithm for the management of bile leak following laparoscopic cholecystectomy. Ann R Coll Surg Engl. 2007;89(1):51–6. https://doi.org/10.1308/003588407X160864. PMID: 17316523 PMCID: PMC1963538.
10. H Pinkas and PG Brady. Biliary leaks after laparoscopic cholecystectomy: time to stent or time to drain. Hepatobiliary Pancreat Dis Int 2008;7(6):628–32. PMID: 19073409.
11. Young ST, Paulson EK, McCann RL, Baker ME. Appearance of oxidized cellulose (Surgicel) on postoperative CT scans: similarity to postoperative abscess. AJR 1993; 160:275–277.
12. Turley BR, Taupmann RE, Johnson PL. Postoperative abscess mimicked by Surgicel. Abdom Imaging 1994; 19:345–346
13. Somani BK, Kasthuri RS, Shave RM, Emtage LA. Surgicel granuloma mimicking a renal tumor. Surgery 2006; 139:451.
14. PD Thurley and R Dhingsa. Laparoscopic cholecystectomy: postoperative imaging. Am J Roentgenol 2008;191:794–801. https://doi.org/10.2214/AJR.07.3485.
15. A Cuschieri, F Dubois, J Mouiel et al. The European experience with laparoscopic cholecystectomy. Am J Surg 161: 385–7. 1991
16. S Connor, OJ Garden. Bile duct injury in the era of laparoscopic cholecystectomy Br J Surg. 2006;93(2):158–68. https://doi.org/10.1002/bjs.5266. PMID: 16432812.
17. P Parrilla, R Robles, E Varo Spanish Liver Transplantation Study Group. et al, Liver transplantation for bile duct injury after open and laparoscopic cholecystectomy Br J Surg. 2014;101(2): 63–68. https://doi.org/10.1002/bjs.9349 PMCID: PMC4253129.
18. DF Mirza, KL Narsimhan, et al. Bile duct injury following laparoscopic cholecystectomy: referral pattern and management. Br J Surg 1997;84(6):786–90. PMID: 9189087.
19. A Nordin, L Halme, H Mäkisalo et al. Management and outcome of major bile duct injuries after laparoscopic cholecystectomy: from therapeutic endoscopy to liver transplantation. Liver Transpl. 2002;8(11):1036–43. https://doi.org/10.1053/jlts.2002.35557. PMID: 12424717
20. Schmidt SC, Settmacher U, Langrehr JM, Neuhaus P. Management and outcome of patients with combined bile duct and hepatic arterial injuries after laparo-

scopic cholecystectomy. Surgery 2004;135(6):613–8. https://doi.org/10.1016/j.surg.2003.11.018.
21. S Adamsen, O H Hansen, P Funch-Jensen et al. Bile duct injury during laparoscopic cholecystectomy: a prospective nationwide series. J Am Coll Surg 1997;184(6):571-8.
22. AM Schreuder, BC Nunez Vas, K A C Booij et al. Optimal timing for surgical reconstruction of bile duct injury: meta-analysis. BJS Open 2020;4(5):776–786. https://doi.org/10.1002/bjs5.50321. PMID: 32852893.
23. R M Hanney, H L Carmalt, N Merrett, N Tait. Vascular injuries during laparoscopy associated with the Hasson technique. J Am Coll Surgeons. 1999; 188(3):337–338. PMID: 10065829 https://doi.org/10.1016/s1072-7515(99)00005-8.
24. M Larobina, P Nottle. Complete evidence regarding major vascular injuries during laparoscopic access. Surg Laparosc Endosc Percutan Tech: 2005;15:119–123. https://doi.org/10.1097/01.sle.0000166967.49274.ca.
25. N Simforoosh, A Basiri, SAM Ziaee, A Tabibi et al. Major vascular injury in laparoscopic urology. JSLS. 2014;18(3):e2014. https://doi.org/10.4293/JSLS.2014.00283 PMCID: PMC4208903 PMID: 25392667.
26. Shu-Hung Chuang and Chih-Sheng Lin: Single-incision laparoscopic surgery for biliary tract disease; World J Gastroenterol. 2016; 22(2): 736–747. https://doi.org/10.3748/wjg.v22.i2.736 PMCID: PMC4716073.
27. L Evers, N Bouvy, D Branje, A Peeters: Single-incision laparoscopic cholecystectomy versus conventional four-port laparoscopic cholecystectomy: a systematic review and meta-analysis; Surg Endosc. 2017;31(9):3437–3448. https://doi.org/10.1007/s00464-016-5381-0 PMCID: PMC5579203.
28. F Fuertes-Guirò and M Girabent-Farrés: Higher cost of single incision laparoscopic cholecystectomy due to longer operating time. A study of opportunity cost based on meta-analysis. G Chir. 2018;39(1):24–34. https://doi.org/10.11138/gchir/2018.39.1.024.
29. Nobumi Tagaya, Keiichi Kubota. Reevaluation of needlescopic surgery. Surg Endosc. 2012;26:137–43. https://doi.org/10.1007/s00464-011-1839-2.PMID: 21789640
30. IG Martin, SPL Dexter, J Marton et al. Fundus-first laparoscopic cholecystectomy. Surg Endosc 9:203–206. (1995). https://doi.org/10.1007/BF00191967
31. Martin IG, Dexter SP, Marton J, Gibson J, Asker J, Firullo A: Fundus-first laparoscopic cholecystectomy. Surg Endosc 1995;9:203–206. https://doi.org/10.1007/BF00191967.
32. Kato K, Matsuda M, Onodera K et al: Laparoscopic cholecystectomy from fundus downward. Surg Laparosc Endosc 1994;4:373–4. https://doi.org/10.1097/00019509-199410000-00012.
33. Uyama I, Iida S, Ogiwara H, Takahara T, Kato Y, Furuta T: Laparoscopic retrograde cholecystectomy (from fundus downward) facilitated by lifting the liver bed up to the diaphragm for inflammatory gallbladder. Surg Laparosc Endosc 1995;5:431–436.
34. Rosenberg J, Leinskold T: Dome down laparoscopic cholecystectomy. Scand J Surg 2004;93:48–51.
35. Tuveri M, Calo PG, Medas F, Tuveri A, Nicolosi A: Limits and advantages of fundus-first laparoscopic cholecystectomy: lessons learned. J Laparoendosc Adv Surg Tech A. 2008;18:69–75.
36. Cengiz Y, Janes A, Grehn A, Israelson LA: Randomized clinical trial of traditional dissection with electrocautery versus ultrasonic fundus-first dissection in laparoscopic cholecystectomy. Br J Surg 2005;92(7): 810–813. https://doi.org/10.1002/bjs.4982.
37. Y Cengiz, M Lund, A Jänes, L Lundell et al. Fundus first as the standard technique for laparoscopic cholecystectomy. Sci Rep. 2019;9:18736. https://doi.org/10.1038/s41598-019-55401-6 PMCID: PMC6904718 PMID: 31822771.
38. Guo-Qian Ding, Wang Cai, Ming-Fang Qin Is intraoperative cholangiography necessary during laparoscopic cholecystectomy for cholelithiasis? World J Gastroenterol. 2015;21(7):2147–2151. https://doi.org/10.3748/wjg.v21.i7.2147 PMCID: PMC4326152.
39. S L Vlek, D A van Dam, S M Rubinstein et al. Biliary tract visualization using near-infrared imaging with indocyanine green during laparoscopic cholecystectomy: results of a systematic review Surg Endosc. 2017;31(7):2731–2742. https://doi.org/10.1007/s00464-016-5318-7 PMCID: PMC5487840.
40. Y Kono, T Ishizawa, K Tani et al. Techniques of fluorescence cholangiography during laparoscopic cholecystectomy for better delineation of the bile duct anatomy. Medicine (Baltimore). 2015;94(25): e1005. https://doi.org/10.1097/MD.0000000000001005. PMCID: PMC4504575.
41. S L Vlek, D A van Dam, S M Rubinstein et al.. Biliary tract visualization using near-infrared imaging with indocyanine green during laparoscopic cholecystectomy: results of a systematic review Surg Endosc. 2017;31(7):2731–2742. https://doi.org/10.1007/s00464-016-5318-7 PMCID: PMC5487840.
42. Nereo Vettoretto, Alberto Arezzo, Federico Famiglietti et al.Laparoscopic-endoscopic rendezvous versus preoperative endoscopic sphincterotomy in people undergoing laparoscopic cholecystectomy for stones in the gallbladder and bile duct Cochrane Database Syst Rev. 2018;2018(4):CD010507. https://doi.org/10.1002/14651858.CD010507.pub2 PMCID: PMC6494553.

References

43. Cuschieri A, Lezoche E, Morino M et al. E.A.E.S. Multicenter prospective randomized trial comparing two-stage vs single-stage management of patients with gallstone disease and ductal calculi. Surg Endosc. 1999;13(10):952–7. https://doi.org/10.1007/s004649901145. PMID: 10526025
44. Sato A, Terashita Y, Mori Y, and Okubo T: Ambulatory laparoscopic cholecystectomy: an audit of day case vs. overnight surgery at a community hospital in Japan. World J Gastrointest Surg. 2012;4(12):296–300. https://doi.org/10.4240/wjgs.v4.i12.296 PMID: 23493831.
45. S Kumar, S Ali, S Ahmad, K Meena and H Chandola. Randomised controlled trial of day-case laparoscopic cholecystectomy vs routine laparoscopic cholecystectomy. Indian J Surg. 2015;77(Suppl 2):520–524. https://doi.org/10.1007/s12262-013-0906-4.
46. Huang X, Feng Y, Huang Z. Complications of laparoscopic cholecystectomy in China: an analysis of 39, 238 cases. Chin Med J (Engl) 1997;110:704–6.
47. Opitz I, Gantert W, Giger U, Kocher T, Krähenbühl L. Bleeding remains a major complication during laparoscopic surgery: analysis of the SALTS database. Langenbecks Arch Surg 2005;390:128–33. https://doi.org/10.1007/s00423-004-0538-z.
48. Lengyel BI, Azagury D, Varban O et al. Laparoscopic cholecystectomy after a quarter century: why do we still convert? Surg Endosc 2012;26:508–13. https://doi.org/10.1007/s00464-011-1909-5.
49. S Suuronen, A Kivivuori, J Tuimala, and H Paajanen. Bleeding complications in cholecystectomy: a register study of over 22, 000 cholecystectomies in Finland. BMC Surg. 2015;15:97. https://doi.org/10.1186/s12893-015-0085-2 PMCID: PMC4535785PMID: 26268709.
50. Thiel, W. Die Konservierung ganzer Leichen in natürlichen Farben. Ann Anat, 174:185–95, 1992.
51. Thiel, W. Ergànzung für die Konservierung ganzer Leichen nach W. Thiel Ann Anat, 184:267–9, 2002.

Part III
Commentaries

Commentaries

Commentary

Desmond H. Birkett

Open cholecystectomy was the only treatment of symptomatic gallstone disease for 100 years, but in the 1980s there were numerous efforts to investigate alternative treatment approaches in an attempt to develop options to an open operation. We tried many of them as they were introduced.

ESWL (extra corporeal shockwave lithotripsy) and dissolution seemed an interesting possibility, but we soon found, as others did, that it was not as effective as originally hoped. It was difficult to fragment the stones effectively and dissolution did not always happen. This was shown to be due to a lack of patency of the cystic duct. Later it was demonstrated by the British/Belgium study which reported stone recurrence was 5% per year with 50% of patients developing recurrent stones at 5 years. To a surgeon it was too slow at achieving results since it often took 18 months to accomplish dissolution and there was a significant recurrence rate.

We then turned to the technique described by Wickham et al. of a minimal access surgical approach to removal of gallstones from the gallbladder. In their technique, they passed a catheter into the gallbladder under radiological control, dilating up the track to permit the placement of a peel-away sheath through which an ureteroscope and an electrolytic hydraulic lithotripter were passed to fragment the stones. With contrast irrigation of saline, the fragments were washed out of the gallbladder. When the gallbladder was free of fragments an 18 Fr Foley catheter was passed through the peel-away sheath into the gallbladder, the balloon blown up and the peel-away sheath removed. The Foley catheter was placed on drainage and removed 2 weeks later. By this time a track had formed preventing leakage into the peritoneal cavity. The wound sealed over the next few days. There were complications of hollow organ injury during the radiological access procedure. Perissat et al. used a similar technique, but they placed the gallbladder catheter and sheath under the direct vision of laparoscopy, which avoided the radiological technique of hollow organ injury. We found this an effective and quick method of removing gallstones with minimal disruption to the patient, but recurrence became a problem and we abandoned it.

Fortunately, around this time there was significant publicity from France about the laparoscopic approach to cholecystectomy. Since this seemed an interesting, and possibly a superior approach to the other techniques, I contacted my friend Jacques Perissat in Bordeaux, and he trained me in the new approach of laparoscopic cholecystectomy.

In 1991, a company developing a 3-D laparoscope approached me and asked me if I was interested in working with them and to use it clinically when fully developed. The laparoscope was a two channel Hopkins rod lens system with a 12 mm outside diameter with two cameras attached to the proximal end. The proximal end was bulky and a little heavy. The images from each camera were alternated on video screen at 120 Hz. One set of images was achieved using both circular polarization in a counterclockwise and clockwise manner.

It gave excellent depth perception and was faster at performing tasks. One senior resident commented, "The era of touch and feel is over," since one could place an instrument in the exact position without having to feel the area first.

In the research laboratory we compared 2D against 3D vision with an experiment of passing a needle and thread through hoops of different sizes placed at different angles and different depths following a set course through the hoops. The exercise was randomized to 2-D and 3-D vision. We found that the exercise was 30% faster in 3-D when each participant's performance was compared in 2D and 3D. Unfortunately, the company folded because of the cumbersome nature of the endoscope with two heavy cameras attached. Now that distal chips are commonplace, 3-D technology is coming back. The endoscopes are much lighter and easier to use. One major issue that has to be overcome is the angulation of the tip of the instrument in 3-D; however, this problem has now been overcome with new technology.

One of the big issues with the move to laparoscopic cholecystectomy was the issue of common duct exploration. Initially we relied on ERCP for the removal of stones. Later, as we became more comfortable performing a laparoscopic cholecystectomy, we started exploring the common bile duct via a choledochotomy. However, with the small ducts we later used the transcystic approach using baskets under fluoroscopy using a choledochoscope. At times cystic duct dilatation became necessary to permit passage of a choledochoscope. The equipment needed for the transcystic approach became an issue because of the specificity of numerous pieces of equipment. It was very important that the scrub nurse and circulating nurse were very familiar with the technology to enable a smooth common duct exploration. However, this became a problem as common duct exploration was only needed in the minority of laparoscopic cholecystectomies and one did not always have the same scrub staff who were familiar with the procedure each time.

I tried single port cholecystectomy in an effort to reduce postoperative pain and secondarily to improve cosmesis. The instruments clashed inside the abdomen and the handles clashed outside the abdomen. It was possible to learn to handle these problems, but the real issue was the loss of triangulation between the endoscope and the instruments, which made it difficult to safely dissect with a 2-D image and loss of triangulation. I, therefore, gave up this approach.

I found that a better approach to reduce postoperative pain and improve cosmesis was to use 3.5 mm trocars in the right upper quadrant and a 5 mm trocar in the epigastrium through which a 5 mm clip applier could be passed. This approach reduced postoperative discomfort considerably because of the reduced abdominal wall trauma from smaller trocars. Gustavo Cavalho, of Recife, Brazil, who designed these small trocars, uses a 3.5 mm trocar in the epigastrium, and instead of a clip applier he ties the cystic duct. This reduces the postoperative discomfort even further.

Although there have been great advances in laparoscopic instruments in the past few decades, there are times when it is necessary to convert to an open operation. This is often a problem for the surgeons brought up after the era of open cholecystectomy. Any conversion to an open operation now in this laparoscopic era is going to mean a difficult open procedure. If not trained in open cholecystectomies, the thought of a difficult cholecystectomy is daunting. The modern surgeon must be prepared to face these difficult dissections like those described by Kehr!

Teaching the Laparoscopic Common Bile Duct Exploration to Acute Care Surgeons

Matthew Bloom

Since their introduction in 2005, several factors have contributed to the adoption of acute care surgery (ACS) services at academic medical centers. These are teams that cover trauma, surgical critical care, and emergency general surgery, and specialize in the treatment of severely ill patients. Around this time, it was recognized that there was a growing population of elderly and increasingly comorbid patients presenting to the emergency room requiring general surgery. Coincidentally, due to improvements in imaging technology, critical care methods, and interventional radiology techniques, the practice of trauma surgery had become less operative resulting in fewer surgical cases. This led to the creation of well-staffed ACS services that were immediately available for, and specialized in the treatment of, acutely ill patients, and which were eager for operative cases. Often staffing emergency departments for both trauma and general surgery call, these teams now end up caring for the majority of acute cholecystitis patients who present to the hospital.

Multiple studies have demonstrated both improved patient outcomes and efficiency of care for patients cared for by ACS services. Large teams of doctors with an immediate around the clock presence coupled with dedicated OR availability help to get patients to the OR faster and to leave the hospital sooner. As a result, a reduction in direct healthcare costs has been repeatedly demonstrated.

In academic centers, these teams typically constitute a significant portion of the resident operative and patient management learning experience. At the same time, many of the attendings who run these services themselves trained in a time when the laparoscopic common bile duct exploration (LCBDE) was not easily performed. This in large part dictates the clinical pathway that their patients will follow. ERCP is heavily relied upon for common duct clearance, either pre- or postoperatively.

But the availability of ERCP is neither immediate nor universal. While some institutions have wonderful access to ERCP and a few in Europe can routinely coordinate ERCP in the OR at the time of surgery, many centers have availability on only certain days of the week, if at all. This reliance upon ERCP adds to patients' length of stay in the hospital, increased anesthetic and procedural risks, and overall healthcare costs.

As an unintended consequence of the shift in rates of gallbladder cases performed laparoscopically, as well as a heightened awareness of missed iatrogenic ductal injury and its significant morbidity, an entire generation of general surgery residents was taught to fear operating upon the common bile duct. Most current graduating residents have performed few, if any, open or laparoscopic operations on this structure. In parallel, the availability of ERCP since 1968 has shunted many ductal procedures out of the operating room to begin with.

And so, as the laparoscopic approach to cholecystectomy gained predominance, the preference for the management of CBD stones shifted to ERCP in the place of surgical exploration. But as confidence and skills in minimally invasive surgery has grown, the trend did not reverse. Now, with the availability of improved instruments, and even disposable ones, the LCBDE becomes an attractive option for surgeons to perform.

An additional benefit of training surgeons to perform LCBDE is its reliance on intraoperative cholangiography (IOC). Performing IOC routinely has been shown to minimize iatrogenic injuries and is the sine qua non for finding the 6–10% of unexpected CBD stones which are incidentally discovered during operation. Not only does routine performance train surgeons for these procedures, but it also trains the OR staff in setting up the equipment and executing these procedures, which makes the entire process smoother and more time efficient, and prepares them for rapid initiation of an LCBDE when indicated.

And it is not too late to "teach old dogs new tricks." Through organized courses that focus specifically on teaching IOC and LCBDE skills to ACS surgeons already performing laparoscopic cholecystectomy, we can train not only this important and overlooked cohort but also expose their trainees to this procedure and further encourage its adoption.

Through these structured courses, ACS attendings are being taught the LCBDE and putting it into practice in their home institutions. We have recently witnessed this precise occurrence. After going through training at our institution, our neighboring academic medical center's ACS service started performing LCBDE on their patients and shortened their patients' length of stay on average by over 1.5 days. This not only provides timelier patient care, it also exposes a new generation of surgeons in training to this procedure and promotes its adoption both within and outside the halls of academia. The delivery of these courses at national meetings remains a high priority.

This is why targeting this particular group of practicing surgeons to learn LCBDE is so essential. Not only will an immediate improvement in patient care be realized, but the dividends in surgical resident education and overall practice adoption will grow exponentially over time.

Commentary: Berci-Greene "No Stones Left Unturned" Kehr Book

L. Michael Brunt

"Where they went, there were no roads" (paraphrased from "Back to the Future")

Drs. George Berci and Rick Greene are to be congratulated for compiling this impressive monograph on the sentinel contributions of Dr. Hans Kehr and the history of biliary surgery from the open through the laparoscopic era. One is immediately struck by the meticulous and careful nature of Kehr's work and the precise documentation of biliary anatomy and pathology through his artistic collaborator. The anatomical illustrations are as apt today as they were over 100 years ago, and this work will be a necessary addition to the library of any serious student of biliary surgery. One can only imagine the end-stage difficulty of many of these cases, and yet operative times were impressively short (35–45 minutes) out of necessity due to the anesthetic techniques and surgical training of that era.

The development of laparoscopic cholecystectomy and the ensuing laparoscopic revolution that transformed surgical practice is one of the most remarkable advances in the history of modern surgery for several reasons: the rapidity with which it occurred; the positive effect it had on virtually every aspect of patient outcomes, return to health and full activity, and morbidity; and the fact that it impacted virtually every surgical discipline. It also spawned a generation of innovative surgeons in both academia and private practice, along with advances in surgical technology and new education and training paradigms that did not exist previously. Perhaps most importantly, these events catalyzed the whole concept of minimally invasive surgery well beyond simply what one could do with a laparoscope and led to a whole new way of thinking about surgical problems beyond traditional definitions of surgical success.

We are indebted to the visionaries and early pioneers who developed, popularized, and promoted acceptance of laparoscopic cholecystectomy: Eric Muhe in Germany and the "Galloscope," Philippe Mouret in France, and Barry McKernan and William Saye who did the first lap chole in the United States in 1988 in Marietta, Georgia [1]. Only two days after McKernan and Saye, Eddie Joe Reddick and Doug Olsen performed a lap chole in Nashville, Tennessee. It was Eddie Joe more than anyone else who popularized this procedure and "trained" numerous surgeons who came to observe him in Nashville, among them Horacio Asbun, 2020-2021 SAGES President, who made multiple trips from California as a resident to learn this new procedure. Eddie Joe unfortunately passed away in 2020, but was truly one of the "unsung" heroes of the early laparoscopic era [2].

Laparoscopic cholecystectomy first received national attention when Jacques Perissat presented a video of his first case at the 1989 SAGES meeting in Louisville, Kentucky. The SAGES leadership immediately recognized the significance and implications of this new approach and came out with a number of position statements regarding who should do this new procedure and established training paradigms for it. Led by George Berci and John Hunter and others, a series of "Train the Trainers" courses were held across the United States to help insure proper training and technique for this new operation [3]. It should be emphasized that none of this could or would have occurred as it did without the pioneering work over decades by George Berci on laparoscopic imaging systems, the Xenon light source, and laparoscopic instrument designed [4].

My own epiphany occurred in November 1989 when Nat Soper presented surgical grand rounds at our institution on gallstone disease and at the very end of his talk, showed a video of the first lap chole he had recently performed in St. Louis at Barnes Hospital. It was as if the veil had lifted on the possibilities, and I became one of the early faculty members at Washington University who scrubbed cases with Dr. Soper to learn how to do lap choles. I, like most of my contemporaries, had no prior experience with laparoscopic surgery, so we had to learn everything from the ground up. We scrubbed with some of the GYN surgeons to become more familiar with techniques for initial laparoscopic access. We also went to the laboratory to develop skills and techniques before performing the first laparoscopic adrenalectomy, splenectomy, Nissen fundoplication, and inguinal hernia repair at our institution which Dr. Soper and I did together. My first SAGES meeting was in 1992 in Washington, DC, where I also first met George Berci. It was the most electrifying surgical meeting I have ever witnessed due to the explosion of innovation and new techniques that was occurring in general surgery.

But back to cholecystectomy. To deal with the demand to learn cholecystectomy in the early 1990s, weekend courses sprang up, and an entire generation of surgeons learned the basic principles of laparoscopic surgery and how to perform an operation they knew so well in a new way. As all are aware, the introduction of LC into clinical practice was associated with a significant increase in the incidence of bile duct injuries (BDI). Thirty years later, bile duct injuries continue to occur at a rate somewhat higher than in the open era and are a significant source of morbidity and, in some cases, mortality for what is an otherwise uncomplicated, outpatient procedure with a rapid recovery and return to health. In 2014, to address this problem SAGES established the Safe Cholecystectomy Task Force with a goal of enhancing a universal culture of safety around cholecystectomy. This task force has undertaken a number of initiatives to help drive the rate of BDI lower. These include carrying out a Delphi process to identify important factors for safety in cholecystectomy which led to the SAGES 6 step program [5, 6]. A series of didactic modules were developed that are available to all surgeons and trainees on the SAGES web site that delves more deeply into the safety aspects and principles of cholecystectomy (available at fesdidactic.org).

In 2018, a multi-society sponsored consensus conference on the prevention of bile duct injury during cholecystectomy was held that addressed 18 key questions on this topic, and guidelines were subsequently published [7]. Taken together, these efforts are important steps in the right direction, but much work remains to be done. Despite the original description of the critical view of safety by Steven Strasburg in 1995 [8], surgeons still incompletely understand and inconsistently apply this method of identification of key ductal structures. The rate of intraoperative imaging is disappointingly low, and surgeons have largely abdicated management of common bile duct stones to the biliary endoscopist. Although new technologies such as near infrared cholangiography hold promise, they are not widely available, nor have they been extensively studied to determine the benefit across the spectrum of patients with gallstone disease. We also lack mechanisms in the United States for tracking bile duct injuries in order to understand the true frequency, patterns, and nature of occurrence. A national system for regionalization of care for patients with bile duct injuries when they occur to specialty centers with an experienced HPB multidisciplinary team would likely improve outcomes and reduce mortality rates and minimize adverse effects on quality of life.

Awareness of the ongoing problem of biliary injuries will not be sufficient to effect change. We must all do our part to educate our colleagues and trainees about best practices for safe cholecystectomy and encourage support for the consensus guidelines. Through these efforts, we can together, I am convinced, push the bile duct injury rate to as close to zero as possible.

The Trajectory of Biliary Surgery: Personal Reflections

Daniel J. Deziel

History and surgery are demarcated by "eras," periods of time defined by their distinctive character, events, and discovery. Since the first known cholecystectomy in 1882, biliary surgery has traversed eras of antisepsis, antibiotics, blood transfusion, and radical oncologic resection into the present era of minimal access and endoscopic technology. Eras are not necessarily confined by hard set boundaries; they are staggered and they overlap as innovation sparks and as prevailing thought transitions at a variable pace.

History and surgery are also distinguished by "generations," by people born and living at the same time, by surgeons trained across a certain period of time or under the philosophy of a particular institution or mentor. The reckoning of progress is inextricably linked to how generations and eras intersect. Some surgical eras have spanned multiple generations with limited change while others have emerged within the span of a single generation or less.

Discovery, innovation, and technological capability are advancing at an increasingly rapid tempo. Surgeons of a "generation" must be able to navigate across "eras." To do this in a way that is nimble, rationale, and responsible is at the crux of how we will assure safe and accountable management for the complete spectrum of our patients' biliary disease and how we will train the coming "generations."

Perhaps my affinity for biliary tract surgery was preordained by my birth at St. Joseph's Hospital in St. Paul, Minnesota, where Justus Ohage performed the first known cholecystectomy in the Western Hemisphere on September 24, 1886 [9]. Perhaps my perception of the current state and trajectory of biliary surgery is balanced by a career that has straddled the eras of open and minimal access operations.

Following excellent residency training in open surgery at Rush, I became the first Gastrointestinal Surgery Fellow at the Lahey Clinic in order to pursue complex pancreaticobiliary surgery under the mentorship of Dr. John Braasch and Dr. Ricardo Rossi. This preceded the existence of any designated HPB fellowships. Returning to Rush as a junior faculty member, I was a primary investigator for a trial of piezoelectric extracorporeal shock wave lithotripsy for gallstones [10]. When laparoscopic cholecystectomy dawned, like many (but not all) early practitioners, I had no prior laparoscopic experience. I was then privileged to train with Dr. Sung Tao Ko and Dr. Mohan Airan, the pioneers of laparoscopic cholecystectomy in Chicago. The lithotripsy experience provided the opportunity to operate on a legion of gallstone patients who had been evaluated for the trial and were eager for the new laparoscopic procedure. Thus, I did the first laparoscopic cholecystectomy operation at Rush on May 23, 1990, and early on was fortunate to develop a sizable experience at an academic center. This was not an unfamiliar tale for some of us.

The era of laparoscopic cholecystectomy exploded unstoppably in a manner without precedent in the history of surgery. Its immediate wake bore the inseparable challenges of training and safety. Early training often featured perfunctory courses offered by industry representatives or for-profit entrepreneurs. Never before had the profession been faced with a need to retrain essentially the entire workforce in the performance of the most common operation in general surgery. The first wide-scale study of complications identified a 0.6% rate of major bile duct injury and included a host of infrequent but potentially catastrophic occurrences [11]. The threat of external regulation by nonmedical entities was palpable.

The Society of American Gastrointestinal and Endoscopic Surgeons (SAGES) stepped into the leadership void early and boldly to remedy the pervasive chaos. The society's first statement on laparoscopic cholecystectomy was issued in October 1989. By May 1990, the time of my first operation, SAGES had released "The Role of Laparoscopic Cholecystectomy—Guidelines for Clinical

Application" and "Granting of Privileges for Laparoscopic General Surgery." To address the need for qualified instructors, a program for "Training the Trainers" was implemented the same year. A process for endorsement of legitimate courses and the first major multi-institutional research study of laparoscopic cholecystectomy followed.

SAGES "Framework for Post-Residency Surgical Education and Training" was a thoroughly conceived document designed to address the critical questions and establish guidelines for postgraduate hands-on training. After years of thought, it was intently honed by brilliant individuals over long hours at Newport Beach in June 1993. I had the privilege to participate in this process and to witness insightful minds dissect the meaning of "preceptor," "proctor," "competence," "proficiency," and "mastery" and to distill principles for postgraduate training that are relevant to this day. Over three decades, SAGES efforts to anchor training and safety in laparoscopic surgery have been a consistent and vital part of the narrative. The establishment of the MIS Fellowship Council, FLS, FES, and FUSE were all initiatives spurred by SAGES. The Safe Cholecystectomy Didactic Modules and the inceptive Multi-society Consensus Conference on the Prevention of Bile Duct Injury During Cholecystectomy with its resultant evidence-based recommendations for safe cholecystectomy highlight more recent endeavors [12, 13].

The safe emergence of minimal access surgery required new technology. In the face of ideologic criticism, SAGES forged a responsible and practical model for cooperation with industry for the development and application of technical innovations for the betterment of patient care. Repurposed and primitive laparoscopic tools have become elegant functional instruments.

During one of our hands-on laparoscopic cholecystectomy courses in 1991, a surgeon, soon to retire, remarked that although he would not be doing laparoscopic surgery himself, he was convinced that soon not only cholecystectomy but most abdominal operations would be done laparoscopically. He said that he would then one day come out of retirement to run courses in open surgery. We chuckled. He was prophetic.

According to the ACGME national case logs, the total number of biliary operations performed by graduating general surgery residents has increased by 74% since 1990 [14]. However, this increase is due solely to laparoscopic cholecystectomy, and all other biliary operations have dramatically declined in frequency. Open cholecystectomy was once the most common resident abdominal operation. Since 2012, the mean number performed has been <10. The mean number of open common bile duct explorations, laparoscopic bile duct explorations, cholecystostomy, sphincteroplasty, or choledochoscopy operations are each <1 and approaching zero. Thirty years ago, my senior faculty mentors would gather to watch me do a laparoscopic cholecystectomy. Now, junior and mid-level faculty surgeons congregate when I do an occasional open common bile duct exploration, complete with fashioning of a Kehr tube.

Residents today are better trained in laparoscopic surgery by faculty surgeons who are better versed than most of us were three decades ago. However, a substitute for experience with difficult open cholecystectomy is not evident. The dictums of safe cholecystectomy, particularly when operative conditions are hazardous, must be ingrained: get experienced help if available, understand the algorithms for secure anatomic identification as set forth in consensus conference recommendations, recognize stopping points and alternatives to complete cholecystectomy. An aborted cholecystectomy operation is retrievable, major bile duct or vascular injury may not be. Correct anatomic identification is requisite to safe cholecystectomy. It is imperative that surgeons know the regularly encountered variations in bile duct and vascular anatomy that have practical significance for safe cholecystectomy. These are not anomalies or aberrations or duplications. These are well-recognized variations that are present with sufficient frequency that they must be anticipated by the watchful surgeon [15]. Indoctrination in the principles of safe cholecystectomy must begin in residency and must be incessant.

The era of surgical management for choledocholithiasis has been slipping away from a generation or more of surgeons. Sometimes things slip because they cannot be effectively grasped, sometimes they are simply released. We have largely entered the time of endoscopic extraction performed by our gastroenterology colleagues since only a minority of surgeons in the United States practice ERCP. This trend was made possible by the expansion of endoscopic capabilities and exacerbated by the reticence of surgeons to pursue laparoscopic common duct exploration. Laparoscopic common bile duct exploration, despite its demonstrated advantages for many patients, and despite available avenues for training, has been approached with reluctance by many surgeons. Various reasons can be given for this: the availability of endoscopic intervention, time, convenience, experience, equipment, skill, reimbursement, and disinterest. Although it will vary by practice setting, open common bile duct exploration has generally become limited to complex cases with stricture, fistula, multiple failed or complicated endoscopic interventions, or otherwise irreparable anatomy. Only if the majority of surgeons who operate on the gallbladder adopt laparoscopic common duct exploration or ERCP into their practice, do I foresee a meaningful resurgence of surgeon treated choledocholithiasis.

I have performed operative imaging of the bile ducts in 92% of the cholecystectomies (open and laparoscopic) that I have done during my attending career. Initially I used intraoperative fluorocholangiography (IOC). For over 20 years, I have routinely performed laparoscopic ultrasonography, supplemented by IOC in certain clinical situations. Thus, I would be considered a "routine" imager. Although selective imaging is well validated, I see an increasing tendency toward more and more "selectivity" to the point that imaging becomes essentially nonexistent. Imaging has the most clinical impact when used for anatomic identification when this is not initially clear by standard dissection and imaging has important yield when there are risk factors for choledocholithiasis. When done routinely, in the absence of other indicators, operative imaging provides valuable experience for trainees to develop and maintain proficiency with the technique so that it can reliably be performed when clinically most important. The disciplines of operative imaging and laparoscopic management of bile duct stones should be integral to resident training.

"The fundamental act of medical care is the assumption of responsibility". So wrote Francis D. Moore M.D. in the introduction to his book, *Metabolic Care of the Surgical Patient* [16]. As surgeons, we have the responsibility to propagate the evaluation and safe application of new technology and methods, to invest in the training of new surgeons and of our practicing colleagues, to implement evidence-based practices, to exemplify dedication to patient care, to commit to self-improvement in our knowledge and technical skills, and to respect the socioeconomic implications of our actions. We will not always make the right decisions at the right time, but our motives need to be clear and our intent honorable. Then generations can safely progress beyond the eras of Kehr and Berci in the unfinished story of biliary surgery.

Commentary

Robert Fitzgibbons and Charles Filipi

It was 1989, and I (RF) was an assistant professor at Creighton University with an established practice after 10 years and a laboratory focused on gallbladder disease. At the time I was studying bile acids in a prairie dog model. Our group had its ears to the ground when the rumblings came out of Nashville that the gallbladder was being removed under laparoscopic guidance. I wondered how this could be possible as my only experience with laparoscopy was watching the gynecologists look down the eyepiece of a laparoscopic telescope with no possibility of assistance because he or she was the only one that could see the operative field. But there was no way to perform a complex operation such as a cholecystectomy without assistance. One of us (CF) at this same time was a surgeon in private practice in Marshalltown, Iowa, and was in discussions with the then Chairman of the Department of Surgery at Creighton, Dr. Tom DeMeester, about joining the department as a full-time faculty member. Dr. Filipi had also heard about the Nashville experience. As it turns out, he had experimented earlier with laparoscopic cholecystectomy in dogs with the help of a gynecologist. The cystic duct and artery were ligated with a Falope Loop (a device used for tubal ligation for sterilization) under guidance with an arthroscopic camera. All of the dogs survived. Nevertheless, Dr. Filipi deemed it not to be feasible primarily because visualization was difficult to maintain due to excessive air leak. Upon hearing about this, Dr. DeMeester immediately had us meet because of mutual interests.

After a short series of meetings, we went to Dr. DeMeester and asked if we could travel to Nashville to see what this was all about. An issue arose, however, when they informed the chairman regarding a charge for going to the operating room to observe the procedure. Initially Dr. DeMeester went into orbit about this, having strong feelings that surgeons have an obligation to share innovations with their fellow surgeons without regard to finances. After all, he had been doing this his whole career. So initially he turned down the request. The next day after he had time to think about it, he came to my (RF) office and told me he was not going to allow his personal feelings to get in the way of the development of his department and that he was going to pay for this visit with departmental funds.

In the spring of 1989, we both traveled to Nashville. At that time, the laser was being used to dissect the gallbladder from the liver bed, almost as if that was the innovation that allowed the procedure to develop. In fact, the name of the operation was "Laser Laparoscopic Cholecystectomy." Upon entering the operating room with Drs. Eddie Reddick and Douglas Olsen performing the procedure, it was immediately obvious that the real breakthrough was the miniature video camera which could be attached to a laparoscope. Now one could perform a complex operation, such as a cholecystectomy with everyone in the operating room seeing the same image on the video screen allowing for adequate assistance. To give Dr. Reddick and Olsen credit, their ingenuity in "jerry rigging" instruments for the procedure was laudable as commercially available instruments did not exist for this new procedure. For example, Dr. Olsen had modified an existing clip applier used for open surgery that could be placed in a laparoscopic cannula without an air leak. Both Dr. Reddick and Olsen were very charming and shared their experience. Dr. Reddick even provided a country western serenade, a hobby that he eventually would pursue professionally.

We returned to Creighton and set up a pig lab and spent 6 months in the lab perfecting the technique. Enough data was obtained to convince the IRB that this could be performed in humans with proper informed consent. The first patient was an employee of the university hospital in late 1989 and the procedure took about 8 hours. Although there was lots of skepticism initially locally, as our experience with the procedure grew, the benefits of minimally invasive surgery became obvious and we were routinely performing five or six cholecystectomies a day.

The academic community at this time was very slow to accept this deviation from conventional surgery. Dr. Nat Soper was the only other academic surgeon who became involved with the procedure initially. In early 1990, I (RF) was asked by Professor E. Moreno Gonzalez from Madrid Spain to share our experience at his highly respected yearly course in general surgery. On May 22, 1990, I (RF) gave a lecture entitled "Cholecystectomy with a laparoscope." There were thousands of attendees from all over Europe. The presentation was well received by the audience, but a panel discussion that followed was more problematic. On that panel were many well-known and highly respected surgeons including Dr. John Najarian from the University of Minnesota and Dr. Seymour Schwartz from the University of Rochester. Dr. Najarian gave an impassioned commentary to the audience saying that only charlatan surgeons in the United States did this operation just to make money; there was no real benefit. Fortunately, most of the other members of the panel, especially Dr. Schwartz, disagreed and felt that this new procedure had significant potential. Ironically after returning home from Madrid, I (RF) received a phone call from Dr. Najarian apologizing for his comments and asking me to come to Minneapolis to teach the surgeons there how to do the operation!

Now there was the daunting task of massive retraining of general surgeons who had no experience with laparoscopy. Dr. George Berci from Los Angeles organized a laboratory session with Drs. Reddick, Eddie Phillips and myself with the express purpose of trying to establish some type of curriculum for orderly dissemination of the technique. The meeting was very successful, but the implementation of the program never really came to fruition because almost immediately, 3-day pig courses sprung up all over the country. Although these courses eventually resulted in the retraining, it was at a cost of a significant increase in cholecystectomy-related visceral and bile duct injuries.

The American College of Surgeons (ACS) recognized that laparoscopic hernia repair would almost certainly follow suit after cholecystectomy given its frequency which rivals cholecystectomy at about 800,000 procedures per year. In an effort to roll out a more orderly training program for laparoscopic herniorrhaphy, I (RF) was asked to join the ACS Committee on Emerging Technology with the express purpose of setting up randomized trials to study this. A grant application was developed looking at laparoscopic inguinal herniorrhaphy versus conventional open herniorrhaphy, but funding was not forthcoming. Only when a third arm, watchful waiting, which could potentially save the healthcare system money, was added was funding successful. The rest of that story is now history. Under Dr. DeMeester's direction an NIH grant application to study laparoscopic cholecystectomy and its risks and benefits was submitted, but eventually not funded.

Jacques Perissat, one of the leaders in minimally invasive surgery in Europe, once wrote, "For a surgeon who performed some of the first laparoscopic cholecystectomies, laparoscopic surgery is undoubtedly the main revolution of the last decade of the 20th century." This quote reflects our feelings as laparoscopy takes its place with other great developments in the history of surgery. We have truly been blessed to be in the right place at the right time. However, although the successes have been rewarding, there have also been the inevitable second thoughts and misgivings along the way when trying to be a pioneer in a field where consequences of our mistakes and the mistakes of those we trained must be borne by our patients. Having said that, laparoscopic cholecystectomy has led the way to a shift to minimally invasive surgery for almost every procedure we perform now as surgeons. This has resulted in a dramatic decrease in the morbidity of our craft. As minimally invasive surgery continues to evolve with better equipment and even robotics, the future seems quite bright.

Laparoscopic Cholecystectomy: At the Beginning...1989–1990

John G. Hunter

In the beginning, it should be noted that open cholecystectomy was the "bread and butter" of most general surgeons in America. While most innovations take 10 years (roughly) to "take hold," the time between the first laparoscopic cholecystectomy (LC) in 1995 and mainstream adoption was only 4–5 years. It was rapidly apparent that the general surgeon who could not take out a gallbladder laparoscopically would be left behind, destined to have their practice limited to hernias and "lumps and bumps." Despite the paucity of randomized clinical trials, the benefits of laparoscopic gallbladder removal were clear to everyone, especially the patients. If a surgeon were to reveal to a patient that they were incapable of performing an LC, the patient usually left to find a surgeon who could perform this procedure.

The Achilles heel of this operation, in the early days, was bile duct injury. The focus of this short piece will be to describe how I became engaged in teaching surgeons safe laparoscopic cholecystectomy, especially focused on prevention of biliary injury. While historical estimates of bile duct injury revealed this complication to occur and approximately 1 to 2 in 1000 gallbladder operations, shortly after laparoscopic cholecystectomy was introduced, common bile duct injuries were occurring almost 10 times more commonly (1%). This created a near epidemic in biliary reconstruction. Clearly there was something wrong with the new operation. Techniques needed to be developed to prevent biliary injury if laparoscopic cholecystectomy was to prove to be a safe operation in the long run.

After talking with students and reviewing published articles on LC technique, it became clear that there were several major issues with how this operation was being performed. The first issue related to the unfamiliarity of most surgeons with biliary anatomy as seen through a video laparoscope. Things were not always as they seemed and the surgeon who injured the common bile duct was often "lost at sea." When they thought they were dissecting out the cystic duct, the identified duct was often the common hepatic duct, leading to its clipping and transection.

In addition to the unfamiliar imaging and anatomic misperception, the technique of laparoscopic gallbladder removal was fundamentally different in that the surgeon did not start by taking the gallbladder down fundus first, as was the standard in open cholecystectomy. The identification of the gallbladder infundibulum as the primary focus of dissection required a different technique. Except in extreme circumstances, LC technique required leaving the gallbladder attached to the liver at the outset of dissection, using the fundus as a handle to elevate the right lobe of the liver to expose the porta hepatis. It was in this setting that the duct which appeared to enter the gallbladder was not the cystic duct, but the common hepatic duct, especially in the setting of significant acute or chronic inflammation.

By adjusting the technique of LC to accentuate five steps in identification of critical anatomy before clips were applied, it allowed the reduction of biliary injury over time. These steps were outlined in an article published in the American Journal of Surgery in 1991 [17]. These steps encouraged the use of an angled laparoscope to provide a variety of perspectives on the gallbladder from the front, from the side and from the back. The second step encouraged the surgeon to elevate the gallbladder fundus sufficiently that the infundibulum was clearly visible superior to the duodenum, and not stuck in the porta hepatis. The third step was lateral retraction of the infundibulum, an attempt to place the cystic duct and common bile duct at right angles or close to that. The fourth step was a circumferential dissection of the infundibulum of the gallbladder at its outlet where the cystic duct originated. By making the gallbladder look like a polyp on a stalk, it was difficult to have anatomic confusion. The fifth and most controversial step was the performance of routine cholangiography. These five steps were termed "Hunter's Principles" by Dr. William Traverso. The first four steps were later compressed into a single statement entitled, "The Critical View of Safety" several years later.

The fifth step, laparoscopic cholangiography—performed routinely—created a great deal of debate. The data were quite clear that the incidence of bile duct injury was 50% less when laparoscopic cholangiogram was performed. Outside of randomized data, there was no way to prove causality. (Note: While randomized trials were attempted, the number of patients that must be randomized to show a difference of 0.03% (3 in 1000) is over 12,000, and thus impractical). Without a randomized clinical trial of adequate size, we could not prove that a cholangiogram prevented bile duct injury, hence the fodder for debate for years to come. Critics of routine cholangiography argued that critical anatomic identification occurs before the presumptive cystic duct is cannulated. Thus, a cholangiogram might identify an injury, but may not prevent it. Perhaps this was not the explanation why BDI was less common with cholangiography than without cholangiography. It was theorized that cholangiograms were performed by the more experienced, better surgeons who were also less likely to injure a common bile duct. And yet a third explanation is possible, that cholangiograms were only done when the anatomy was clear and inflammation was minimal. In this setting, a biliary injury would be expected to be less frequent. Be that as it may, it was probably not the data that swung the argument one way or another but the sense that surgeons did not want to be bothered with the time commitment and the technical difficulty of performing a cholangiogram when the anatomy was clear and the likelihood of a bile duct stone was low.

The standard of care today does not require routine cholangiography as long as the first four of "Hunter's principles" are performed and the "critical view" is attained. Whether or not routine cholangiography prevents injury, few would argue against having this technique in a surgeon's toolkit, so that they may use it as needed to confirm anatomy or search for suspected CBD stones. In a teaching institution, it is imperative that general surgery residents are trained in the techniques of cholangiography. While the incidence of laparoscopic biliary injury is now close to that of open surgery, injuries are still created by experienced as well as inexperienced laparoscopic surgeons. When a surgeon is unable to perform the first four steps in "Hunter's Principles" to make the gallbladder look like a polyp on a stalk (and obtain the critical view), it is probably time to call in a colleague to help them through the operation. If a colleague is unavailable or similarly challenged by the anatomy, it is time to convert to open cholecystectomy.

In conclusion, laparoscopic cholecystectomy was a revolutionary operation that disrupted the status quo in general surgery. The torch was carried forward by innovative surgeons of all ages and within a very short window of time LC became the standard of care for symptomatic gallstone disease. Familiarity with cholangiography, developed by many through its routine application, allows the surgeon confidence to perform a laparoscopic bile duct exploration when needed and feel confident in the identification of biliary anatomy. If a surgeon is not familiar with laparoscopic cholangiography, their only default will be to refer patients for postoperative ERCP when bile duct stones are suspected. This is a bit unfortunate as there is no better access to the common bile duct to remove stones than the access that is gained through the cystic duct during laparoscopic cholecystectomy, especially after stone passage.

Personal Perspective/Experience—In This Surgical Space

Joseph B. Petelin

Having been a surgeon for over 40 years and having started my laparoscopic studies in the late 1980s, performing my first laparoscopic cholecystectomy in September 1989, and first laparoscopic common bile duct exploration in the spring of 1990, I have been fortunate to have successfully performed over 6000 laparoscopic cholecystectomies, over 6000 laparoscopic intraoperative cholangiograms (IOCs), and over 600 laparoscopic common bile duct explorations. As a founding member of the "Fellowship Council" I have trained numerous surgeons and fellows over the past 30 years. I have performed over 20,000 laparoscopic cases. While my practice is heavily focused on biliary tract disease, I have performed all types of advanced laparoscopic procedures, including the world's first laparoscopic splenectomy and the first laparoscopic adrenalectomy in 1990, thousands of laparoscopic colectomies, laparoscopic anti-reflux procedures, etc. In 1991, I hosted one of the first international symposia on Minimal Access Surgery in Kansas City—a term I coined at that time. (I later preferred to refer to it as *Minimally Invasive Surgery*—refining the focus to its effects on *patients*, not surgical techniques.)

Historical Context: The Early Pioneers

Drs. Berci and Greene have done a remarkable job of reviewing the early history of the surgical treatment of benign biliary tract disease, highlighting the innovation and rigor that Professor Kehr and others brought to the field.

Recent Developments and We "Late Comers"

It would appear that the *rate* of change in surgical experience and technology has continued to increase over the past 100+ years—not unlike (but much slower than) Moore's Law regarding the rate of change in computing power in the silicon space. Nevertheless, there are common threads that underlie the work that these early "pioneers" accomplished and that have been "re-sewn" over the past three decades.

Convergence of Disciplines

One of these interesting features of this development involves the "convergence of disciplines." Note that Professor Kehr incorporated the expertise of someone in a different discipline, an artist, to document the details of surgical procedures; it was their late afternoon discussions that had an added benefit. It taught Mr. Frohse about surgery, and their collaboration enhanced Kehr's performance of the procedures. This obviously facilitated the education of other surgeons. Note how the more recent convergence of our surgical discipline with the technological disciplines enabled the advancements of laparoscopic surgery and enhanced the ability to teach others about new techniques in vivid detail—think Berci's rod and lens scopes adapted from Hopkins, teaching scopes with a separate eye-piece, clip appliers, video-laparoscopes, flexible choledochoscopes, etc. How did this happen?

Disruptive Technologies

There came …computers, and the technology to put a CCD (charged coupled device) (i.e., video camera) on a chip! It seemed like magic that a surgeon could share with others in the room what he or she was seeing in the abdomen through a 10 mm port.

The philosopher Arthur Clarke once presented an idea about technology:

> *Any sufficiently advanced technology is indistinguishable from magic.* —Arthur C. Clarke, *Profiles of the Future: An Inquiry into the Limits of the Possible*

Apply this thought to the conventional academic surgical establishment in the 1990s and its reluctance to accept minimally invasive surgery as anything but a gimmick—"magic"! Nevertheless, the world was changing—an inflection point had occurred.

That concept was clearly described in 1996 by Andy Grove, past founder and CEO of Intel, in his most famous book entitled *Only the Paranoid Survive*. In that book he described "strategic inflection points" in business and technology. His company had been wildly successful and those who were responsible for achieving it were "wed" to the technology that made Intel successful. He described how the company almost missed the strategic inflection point in computer technology by defending the existing technology that had gotten them to that point. It took new thinking and new technology to grow. He and the company had only dealt with and communicated with other companies that used their products to *make* computers—not with the end user—their real client who *used* the computers. Sound familiar? Consider these quotes from his book and consider applying them to our field of surgery, then read on:

> *In short, strategic inflection points are about fundamental change in any business, technological or not*
> *Businesses fail either because they leave their customers or because their customers leave them!*
> *The person who is the star of a previous era is often the last one to adapt to change, the last one to yield to logic of a strategic inflection point and tends to fall harder than most.*
> *People in the trenches are usually in touch with impending changes early*
> —Andrew S. Grove, *Only the Paranoid Survive*

Current State

Inflection point considerations can certainly be applied to our surgical space. Note how open cholecystostomy was initially preferred over the newer open cholecystectomy in those early days—over a century ago. Seems illogical for us today that surgeons would have assumed that idea back then—just as it seems illogical that many academic surgeons assumed that open cholecystectomy would never be replaced by this new gimmick, "lap chole," in the early 1990s. Many academic surgeons in the establishment were accustomed to writing papers, pontificating at podiums and only discussing surgery with their peers as their main audience, despite the fact that they were operating on their real *end user*—their patients. They missed the inflection point! (If you get a chance to read just the first 100 pages of Grove's book, the similarities to the current state of surgery are glaring!)

And so grew the relatively untamed "weekend course"—mostly in the private sector (the "trenches"). Unfortunately, only a handful of devoted "private" surgeons, who maintained the rigors and surgical principles learned in open surgery in their courses, produced high quality courses. Space does not provide a thorough discussion of the many reasons for this development, but suffice it to say that patients realized the benefits of this new approach (just as computer "geeks" realized that they were the real consumers of Intel's products), patients demanded the new surgery, and the academic surgical establishment missed the inflection point. (Similarity to Intel in 1994!)

Surgical Training

I am not sure at all that we as a profession have learned as much as we should have from the past—and there are many reasons for that. I am told that surgical residents are generally performing a fair number of laparoscopic cholecystectomies but very few are being trained to perform IOC, and even fewer have any experience with laparoscopic common bile duct exploration (LCDE). It is also not clear to me whether many, if not most, of our surgical educators have expertise in LCDE. It seems that general surgeons have abandoned the common bile duct, yielding it to our GI colleagues (who do a great job). Remember that Traverso et al. [18] have documented that adding ERCP/S to laparoscopic cholecystectomy significantly increases the cost and adds potential morbidity to the treatment of patients with common duct stones—even in the hands of an expert endoscopist. Interestingly, one of the younger GI doctors at my institution told me that he and most GI residents were never to perform ERCP, and that it was being reserved for certain fellows. So, are we headed for a perfect storm?

Final and Future Thoughts

As I understand it, surgery for biliary tract pathology is only a few hundred years old. I would guess that we are still in the infancy or adolescence of this field. Great improvements have been made in treating these patients, especially with the recent introduction of laparoscopic surgery, but maybe as Longmire envisioned, we will abandon what we know today as the best surgery for biliary tract problems with the advent of advanced technology that we cannot even imagine at this time. And yes, as someone with over three decades of experience in this field, I *don't* see that so-called robotic surgery at its current state, is it! — but that is a long difficult discussion that might reveal the Emperor's Clothes and is not indicated here.

I do have concern that we as surgeons are abrogating our responsibility to treat benign biliary tract disease, potentially putting our patients at more risk. As Jacques Perissat suggested in 1994:

"We must move towards a management policy using today's technology, which prevents patients from needing a dangerous and debilitating second operation if there is a stone left in the CBD" [19]. In surgical training we were always taught to perform the best operation for the patient, for the appropriate indication, at the right time, in the most efficient and cost-effective manner. It seems to me that laparoscopic cholecystectomy with IOC, and LCDE when necessary, is the only approach for patients with CBD stones that satisfies those criteria at this time.

Yes, I know it is difficult…but surgeons are not supposed to be afraid of what is difficult…

This quote from another famous philosopher seems appropriate:

Those who cannot remember the past are condemned to repeat it. —George Santayana, *The Life of Reason*, 1905.

I believe, and hope, that the next "inflection point" in surgery is near…

Each Major Advance in Biliary Surgery Needed a New Way of Teaching

Edward H. Phillips

The surgical management of biliary disease has undergone four major changes since the early 1800s. Prior to 1867, lancing an abdominal wall boil and creating a biliary cutaneous fistula was the only surgical treatment for those patients lucky enough to survive up until that point. Theodore Kocher (1841–1917), the famous Swiss surgeon, tried to create a cholo-cutaneous fistula and performed his first cholecystotomy in 1854 while Bobbs performed the first in the USA in 1867. While a cholecystotomy was thought to be experimental and dangerous, Karl Langenbuch (1846–1901) went even further and performed the first cholecystectomy in 1882. He treated common bile duct stones by milking them back into the gallbladder. Open surgery was a major advance but not without significant risks and challenges. It required an increased reliance on visual inspection and less reliance on tactile sensation. It required the need for light, exposure, a skilled assistant, anesthesia, antisepsis, and a hospital operating room. Of course, initially there was increased mortality due to bleeding, infection, and anesthetic complications inherent in "big" incision surgery. Advances progressed rapidly. In 1889, the first choledochotomies were being reported by Abbe in New York, Thornton in London, Courvoisier in Switzerland, and Kehr in Germany. In 1899, William Halsted performed the first choledocho-duodenostomy. These surgeons, teaching by apprenticeship and publication of their work, also experienced something in common—they faced harsh criticism from their colleagues for embarking on dangerous and unproven operations.

My fascination with the biliary tree began when I first met George Berci. I was a surgical resident at LA County-USC Medical Center in 1976 when he introduced the rigid choledochoscope as a visiting lecturer. Three years later, I went into practice at Cedars-Sinai Medical Center in Los Angeles where George was on faculty. But in retrospect, my circuitous journey to laparoscopic cholecystectomy occurred a few years later when Dr. Bernie Fisher published the results of a trial showing equivalent survival between mastectomy and breast-preserving surgery followed by radiation. Dr. Fisher ultimately prevailed against fierce resistance, the loss of his job as Chair and the animosity of his colleagues that is often directed at disruptive innovators. As Machiavelli said, "The innovator makes enemies of all those who prospered under the old order and only lukewarm support is forthcoming from those who would prosper under the new."

I believed Dr. Fisher's data and was an early adopter of breast preserving surgery. Each consult was an emotional roller coaster. I often stayed late into the night trying to help patients and their families with such an emotionally charged decision: mastectomy or lumpectomy. It was also my first experience getting pushback from my colleagues. I soon learned firsthand what Fisher was up against. It was an emotionally exhausting time for me, and maybe a dose of research on an exciting project would rejuvenate me. Enter Dr. George Berci who was Primary Investigator on the Siemens trial for extracorporeal lithotripsy for gallstones (circa 1984). This was a trial that changed my life. The Siemens protocol required a surgeon to evaluate and be on call for each participant. When Dr. Berci asked me to be that surgeon, I un-enthusiastically said "yes." I was truly shocked when so many people enrolled in the trial. I thought an open chole was a great operation. So why were not these people excited to have a cholecystectomy? I learned that they had seen their parents and/or grandparents suffering with chronic pain, incisional hernias, bile fistulae, and postoperative mortality.

This was a light bulb moment I decided to go into the animal lab and develop a better way to perform a cholecystectomy occurred . At this point, I have to thank the late Dr. Leon Morgenstern, the Director of Surgery at Cedars and a great figure in American surgery. He gave me the opportunity to pursue something he thought was dangerous and would not work. Fortunately, all the elements needed to take an idea to reality were available at Cedars-Sinai Medical Center: it had a large animal lab where I could experiment on pigs and learn from my mistakes, it had relationships with industry including Karl Storz Endoscopy that supplied the laparoscopic equipment for the lab and it had George Berci an innovator in all things endoscopic. There were several technical challenges to overcome: exposure of the gallbladder which required designing better graspers. It needed better tools for dissection: an instrument that could dissect and provide hemostasis was needed, a hook cautery was developed and ultimately the Probe Plus (Ethicon EndoSurgery) with cautery, suction, and irrigation. Finally, ligation of the cystic duct and artery was performed with suture and extracorporeal knot tying. An endoscopic clip applier had to be developed. Next was practice, practice, practice. By early 1988, we were ready to do a lap chole on a human patient. Unfortunately, Dr. Morgenstern did not agree. He thought it was too dangerous.

We were stymied until we heard a few other surgeons were doing lap choles around the world. The closest was Dr. Eddie joe Reddick in Nashville working with William Saye. We were not aware of Eric Mühe's work nor how he lost his license for performing lap choles. Dr. Berci and I got on a plane and went to watch Dr. Reddick perform a lap chole using the CO_2 laser for dissection. The surgical technique was similar to ours but we used hook electrocautery. After returning to Cedars with his video, we were able to get IRB permission for a 20-patient pilot study. It was not easy to get the first patient to consent. It took 4 months. Finally, a surgery was scheduled in October 1989. It took 3 ½ hours. It went well and the patient did fantastically well.. The difference between a laparoscopic and an open chole was dramatic. No randomized control trials were necessary to convince that laparoscopic surgery was the future. But like Bernie Fisher's and Eric Muhe's experience as well as the experience of early biliary surgeons, being an innovator always has its obstacles: competitors limited my surgical privileges.

Dr. Berci correctly thought that would change if we taught all 60 of the general surgeons on staff how to perform lap choles. So we geared up to give weekend courses in the lab. Initially I had incorrectly assumed we would teach lap chole the same way we taught residents "open" cholecystectomy: see one, do one, teach one. But this was such a new way of operating. The old way of teaching would not suffice. I had never attended, let alone organized a hands-on course with lap trainers and pigs, but with George Berci's help, the support of our lab assistant, Leon Dayhovsky, and my partners Brendan Carrol and Moses Fallas, the resources of Cedars and instrumentation from Karl Storz and Ethicon EndoSurgery, we started teaching the teachers and then, community surgeons.

The laparoscopic revolution was the beginning of my experience in postgraduate surgical education. The demand for courses was tremendous but not all courses were created equal. Facebook's original motto was to "move fast and break things," and Silicon valley's mantra is to "fail fast and fail often." However, this will not cut it with our patients' lives at stake. Even if the courses were good, many surgeons began performing laparoscopic cholecystectomies after a single weekend course. As feared, complications were occurring at an alarming frequency. Ultimately, SAGES stepped up and took the lead setting standards and certifying courses.

It became immediately apparent that a technique to remove common duct stones encountered during lap chole was needed. Many surgeons were relying on ERCP/ES but not without complications of stricture, perforation, and pancreatitis—especially on young patients with small ducts. Leon Dayhovsky had been a urology technician and he taught me urologic techniques for removing ureteral stones. We tried ampullary balloon dilation and lavage, laser and electrohydraulic lithotripsy via the ureteroscope, and fluoroscopic wire basket stone retrieval. In December 1989, I began using sequential bougies (and later radial dilating balloons) to dilate the cystic duct, a ureteroscope, and wire basket to retrieve stones in favorable cases and later, choledochotomy in dilated common ducts which led to adding laparoscopic suturing and intracorporeal knot tying to our skill set.

Dr. Berci, myself, and others tried to encourage surgeons to utilize cholangiography, not only to identify stones and confirm anatomy but also to identify bile duct injuries during cholecystectomy so that they could be repaired promptly and reduce the sequelae. Even then, some surgeons did not identify injuries on cholangiograms as they were not familiar with reading cholangiograms. Since most surgeons could not or did not want to remove bile duct stones laparoscopically, intraoperative cholangiograms were not performed except by a relatively small group of experts. Because bile duct injuries persist even 30 years since the introduction of laparoscopic cholecystectomy, SAGES initiated a Safe Cholecystectomy program. As surgeons teaching cholecystectomy, our work is not done.

But what of the future? The future is here—robotic cholecystectomy. In 2020, 25% of academic centers on the west coast of the United States are routinely performing robotic cholecystectomies and that number is increasing. Even though tactile sensation is lost, the robotic technique has superior visualization and a skilled assistant, PA, or nurse is not really needed. The surgeon can retract for themselves while sitting at an ergonomic console. And with any new technology, a new way of teaching is needed. Robotic surgery has a teaching console which allows the teacher to safely control the student and point out key steps and anatomy. It is a great teaching tool but expensive and not as available as a lap trainer had been. Unfortunately, as more and more residents are training in robotic surgery, the number of robotic cholecystectomies is increasing while intraoperative cholangiograms are decreasing even more. To perform a cholangiogram, it takes time to scrub back in, put a catheter percutaneously through the abdominal wall, insert it in into the cystic duct, and clip it there. The robot needs to be de-coupled from the working ports so a fluoroscopy machine can be brought in to perform the cholangiogram. It is not going to happen except in very selected cases. It takes too much time.

Another challenge to surgical bile duct exploration is the change occurring in emergency surgery. Acute care surgeons are performing most of the emergency surgery in urban centers and they are teaching the residents emergency cholecystectomies. Most acute care surgeons have not been trained in laparoscopic common duct exploration. These changes have resulted in the trend that common duct explorations are only being performed on patients who have had gastric bypasses or complicated stone disease. Increasingly, these are being performed by hepatobiliary surgeons many of whom have also not been trained in techniques of bile duct exploration, let alone endoscopic techniques. However, I believe in the future robotic biliary surgery will be augmented by artificial intelligence which will alert the surgeon to anatomic variants making the operation safer. Robotic endoscopic ultrasound will help identify not only the anatomy, but also bile duct stones. Robotic-guided bile duct endoscopy and stone removal, therefore, will bring the bile duct back into the surgeon's realm.

Biliary Surgery: A Story of Innovation and Change

Jeffrey L. Ponsky

The gallbladder and biliary tree have long been a focus of fascination for physicians.

Early surgeons approached the gallbladder with some caution as they were unsure if one could survive without it. The first interventions in this area included draining the obstructed gallbladder, then later, opening it and removing the stones. In Berlin, in 1882, Carl Langenbuch demonstrated the temerity to remove the organ. Then followed a century of refinement and expansion of surgical approaches to the biliary tree. In addition to cholecystectomy for cholecystolithiasis, surgeons developed great skill and confidence in operating upon the common bile duct, for treatment of choledocholithiasis and also for other benign and malignant maladies.

Surgery upon the biliary tree could be easy and rapid, but frequently proved challenging and complicated. Inflammation or anatomic variation in biliary anatomy could make interventions difficult and occasionally lead to dire complications. Compulsive attention to details of operative technique and identification of anatomy became hallmarks of biliary surgery. By the middle of the twentieth century, general surgeons became quite comfortable with the operative therapy of biliary lithiasis. Operations on the common bile duct were quite routine and highly successful. The incidence of bile duct injury was exceedingly low.

Other methods of therapy for biliary stones emerged in the 1970s and 1980s. These included endoscopic retrograde cholangiopancreatography (ERCP) and extracorporeal shockwave lithotripsy (ESWL). ERCP offered a means to examine the bile duct, identify pathology, and remove bile duct stones by incising the ampulla of Vater and passing a variety of instrumentation up the duct to remove the stones. This method became extremely popular and highly successful in treating choledocholithiasis but carried its own risk of complications. It did not address gallbladder stones. ESWL used high-frequency sound waves to fracture stones. Although highly successful in the therapy of kidney stones, and initially thought to be an alternative to cholecystectomy for gallstones, the latter did not prove to be true.

Perhaps the most revolutionary advance in the recent history of biliary surgery was the development of laparoscopic cholecystectomy. This method, first performed in Germany in 1985, fired the imaginations of surgeons throughout the world and was rapidly embraced by the public. It provided for a means of removing the gallbladder (and eventually almost every other organ) in a minimally invasive way with reduced morbidity. While a number of surgeons became comfortable exploring the common bile duct, either through the cystic duct or by direct laparoscopic choledochotomy, most deferred to ERCP, either pre- or postoperatively to manage stones in the bile duct. The frequency of intraoperative cholangiography remained low.

While this approach was mostly effective, there was an added cost and morbidity attendant to the added ERCP.

Recent innovations in endoscopic technology have led to the development of very high-quality small caliber choledochoscopes which can be passed through the cystic duct and facilitate stone extraction from the common duct. Unfortunately, training in this technique has not kept pace with innovation. Surgical residency programs have offered little exposure to common bile duct exploration. Specialty societies such as SAGES (Society of American Gastrointestinal and Endoscopic Surgeons) and individual surgeons such as the authors of this monograph have emphasized the importance of training surgeons in these techniques, and offered courses and training materials to support these efforts.

Innovation in the area of biliary surgery has not ceased. In the early part of the twenty-first century a new concept called NOTES (Natural Orifice Translumenal Endoscopic Surgery) was introduced. This idea excited surgeons and gastroenterologists throughout the world. An early goal of this project was to create a means of performing transgastric cholecystectomy.

Although some of these procedures were successfully performed, they failed to achieve wide acceptance due to technological and conceptual shortfalls. In addition, none of these procedures addressed common bile duct stones. Thus, for the present, the method has been mostly abandoned.

More recent innovations in attacking biliary lithiasis have involved the therapeutic use of endoscopic ultrasound and endoscopic stent technology. In select cases, the gallbladder can be visualized via the stomach or duodenum with endoscopic ultrasound. A wire is passed across the intestinal wall into the adjacent gallbladder and a self-expanding stent is passed across the walls into the gallbladder. The edges of the stent turn back to create a tight anastomosis and an endoscope may be passed into the gallbladder and the stones extracted into the Intestinal lumen: A permanent cholecysto-enteric anastomosis is thus created.

These new innovations are exciting and, in some cases, transformative, as was laparoscopic cholecystectomy, and indeed, open cholecystectomy itself. However, in the excitement to create new methodology and innovation, the issue of the common bile duct is usually overlooked. Removal of stones therein relegated to treatment by ERCP. While this is certainly effective in most cases, it is clear that modern surgeons have relinquished their dominance in the treatment of choledocholithiasis to the endoscopist. The average general surgeon of today is uncomfortable in the management of common duct stones.

The practice of biliary surgery in the future will continue to evolve as new technologies and expertise develop. Innovation will continue to occur, and patients will benefit as robotics and artificial intelligence are integrated into biliary therapy. It is important, however, for surgical training programs to emphasize expertise in the management of common duct pathology. These therapies were developed by surgeons and surgeons of the future must continue to own this space.

Commentary

Walter J. Pories

My worst case as a chief resident at the University of Rochester was a Puerto Rican father of eight who presented with jaundice and abdominal pain. On exploration through a long right upper quadrant incision, I encountered a large common duct with impacted stones that I could not budge. We squinted through a small, monocular choledochoscope but could not see much and finally dislodged the offending rock with difficulty. He died 3 days later of hemorrhagic pancreatitis, no doubt due to my excessive manipulations. Even now, 58 years later, I still rue this death.

Today, because of George, surgeons are far more capable of managing these cases with excellent outcomes, through little incisions, with precision. Because of his inventions of new instruments, his adaptation of optics into medical practice, his pursuit of laparoscopy and thoracoscopy, we no longer need to squint through foggy tubes with our heads almost into the wound. Due to his vision, his adaptation of tiny cameras, we can now observe our movements on large monitors in two dimensions, in color. We can record the procedures and use these videos for teaching, not only for students but for ourselves. Surgery can even be directed from another part of the globe and, perhaps soon, during interplanetary travel. Nor were his contributions limited to explorations of the large cavities. He also made it possible to traverse the entire colon, much of the foregut and the entire tracheobronchial tree with ease and certainty, allowing not only visualization but also diagnosis, resection of lesions, and even curative removal of tumors. His maturation of colonoscopy, allowing definitive safe screening, alone has saved countless lives.

One can only wonder, as he sits in his apartment in Los Angeles isolated by the pandemic, what new ideas he has in store for us. I asked him recently to share his vision of the future but he was reticent, a response I took to mean that he was already off on another breakthrough, perhaps the design of small, insect-like robots, swallowed in a capsule, that escaped from that container into the stomach, moved through the gastric wall into the abdominal cavity, carried out the destruction of tumors or clearing of lesions, returning into the bowel to be discharged at a later time, perhaps with a small specimen of the lesion in another retrievable capsule. Stay tuned.

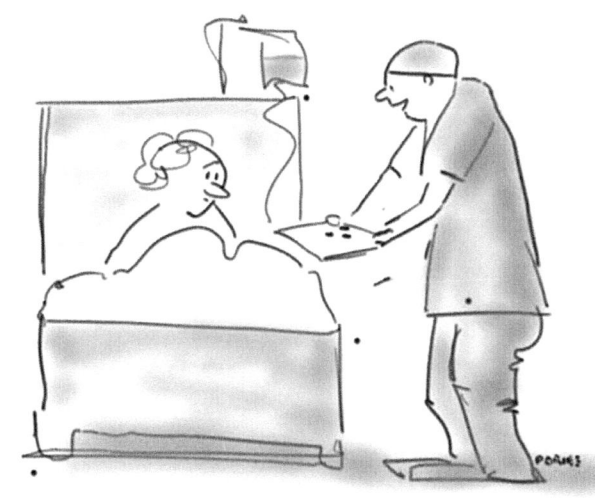

"I know they look like insects but these are the little robots that we'll put in your tiny incisions so they can do the operation."

This translation of the work of Hans Kehr not only is a total pivot into the past but indicates how far we have come. The image of Kehr performing a cholecystectomy in about 1900 brings it home. Note the lack of masks, caps, gloves, and the surgeon, with bare hands, reaching up into the gallbladder fossa with his left hand.

Berci's elegant translation also allows us to appreciate the art of medical illustration. As a medical illustrator, I have long been fascinated by the curious history of this invaluable aid to medical education. Accurate anatomy, displayed in statues and friezes, was prized by the ancient Greeks and Romans, but fell in disfavor in the Church. In the eleventh and thirteenth centuries papal encyclicals emphasized the teaching that existence on this earth was a test to determine if a sinner was fit to enter heaven. Based on that belief, they forbade monks from serving as physicians, but allowed nuns to continue to provide palliative care. Part of those pronouncements also led to the prohibition of anatomic dissections and medical illustration. An exception was finally granted to artists, a ruling that led to DaVinci's production of the finest anatomic drawings of his time.

Medical illustration returned in the American Civil War with a series of remarkable watercolors by surgeons. At the turn of the century, German surgeons, including Kehr, helped to promote medical illustration for teaching purposes. It was not until 1884, with the arrival of Max Broedel at Johns Hopkins that the discipline flourished in the United States.

First, George Berci led us into the future. Now with this remarkable translation of the book by Hans Kehr, he guides us into the past. Enjoy the excerpts from Kehr's remarkable publication and join me in reflecting how far our field has come.

For Me, It Started with Diagnostic Laparoscopy

Barry Salky

I remember, like yesterday, the conversation I had with George Berci in the mid-1980s while attending a diagnostic laparoscopy course in Florida. The question had to do with using diagnostic laparoscopy for retroperitoneal pathology.

A little bit of history is appropriate here. When I finished my surgical training in 1979 (no CT or MRI and just at the infancy of sonography), I was introduced to diagnostic laparoscopy as a way to detail problems in the abdomen. I learned from H. Worth Boyce, MD, at the University of South Florida. He taught me the technique of introducing the laparoscope under local anesthesia. N_2O was the preferred insufflation gas, not CO_2 as is used today. It was eye opening for me. I was amazed at how this simple technique could change the clinical course for so many people. There were very few general surgeons versed in this technique in the United States (George Berci was one!). Being a general surgeon, I was always interested in the therapeutic possibilities of laparoscopy more so than its diagnostic capabilities. Then, laparoscopic cholecystectomy was introduced. I learned the technique from Professors Perissat and Dubois in late 1989. Clearly, this was a game changer for all surgeons.

I remember well the push back from both academia and private practice surgeons, both for different reasons. Academic pushback had to do more with changing the surgical paradigm, while many private practice surgeons saw this as an economic assault. It was a difficult time in the early 1990s for advancement of laparoscopic cholecystectomy. I was trained in routine (open) cholangiography, so adding that to lap chole was not difficult for me. However, it was difficult for many surgeons, and I believe, it was key to the increase in common bile duct injuries with lap chole. As I practiced in New York City at The Mount Sinai Hospital, the New York State Health Department's scathing report on common bile duct injuries is still fresh in my mind. While the incidence of bile duct injuries in lap chole has come down, it is still higher than open cholecystectomy historically.

Training was (and still is!) a major issue in 1990, and it was clearly all over the place. Some private practice surgeons saw this as an economic tsunami. Many medical device manufacturers were scrambling to get into the field. Many general surgeons were clamoring to learn the technique. It was truly the surgical "wild west" in the 1990s. The patients who needed cholecystectomy only wanted it done laparoscopically. In 1990, it was not uncommon to have five laparoscopic cholecystectomies a day on my operative schedule, and I operated 3 days a week! One thing was clear to me back then: laparoscopic cholecystectomy was going to bring a revolution to general surgery. Cholecystectomy was just the start. It was clear that innovation was going to disrupt general surgery. The difference in recovery was just as dramatic as the difference in scar formation from what general surgeons were trained to expect. That is just as true today as it was then. A good example of this is colon and rectal surgery. There is debate among surgeons if intracorporeal anastomosis has advantages over extracorporeal techniques. Both require training, but intracorporeal requires a more advanced skill set in suturing. Smaller incisions (or even no abdominal incision) are possible with intracorporeal techniques, all to the patient advantage.

Of all the surgical societies in the United States, it was the Society of American Gastrointestinal and Endoscopic Surgeons (SAGES) that recognized a revolution in surgery was coming. To its credit, SAGES promoted proper, organized training in laparoscopic cholecystectomy. It issued guidelines so needed by patients and surgeons. SAGES's stature in American surgery soared dramatically (appropriately so) in its activities related to the laparoscopic revolution. There were many in the SAGES organization that were responsible for this, including the authors of this book. SAGES continues to focus on minimally invasive surgery in all its aspects for general surgeons, and laparoscopic cholecystectomy continues to be part of it. SAFE cholecystectomy is a relatively new initiative promoted by SAGES.

Where will minimally invasive surgery go next? How will it impact patients, surgeons, and the medical economy in general? I wish I had the answer to those questions, but I am sure that surgery will change, just as it did in late 1989 and early 1990. Robotics have made a strong push into this arena, but exactly what and how has not been determined. The good news is that we learned a lot from the early days of laparoscopic cholecystectomy. Patient safety and clinical effectiveness are the two most important components of the next revolution. SAGES is continuing to keep those parameters front and center of their credo. Science must rule the day in surgery, and I am looking forward to where it will take us. That does not mean that innovation has to be stifled. It just means that innovation has to be properly set up so that we and our patients get the correct answers. This very much includes robotics and its role in minimally invasive surgery.

Commentary

Jozsef Sandor

In 1909, Sir Granville E. Smith in London presented a mummy as a gift to the Royal College of Surgeons. Princess Amenen's mummy originated from the twenty-first dynasty. A careful examination of the remnants of viscera revealed an enlarged gallbladder which contained 30 gallstones. This finding from 1500 BC was evidence of mankind's suffering from gallstone disease for more than 3000 years.

There was no solution to get rid of this disease: only those could survive the complications of inflamed gallbladder who were lucky to develop a fistula from the gallbladder to the abdominal wall through which gallstones and bile were passing during their life. The first successful surgical intervention—cholecystostomy—was performed by J.S. Bobbs in 1867 (with anesthesia) in Indianapolis on the third floor of a drugstore. This was a successful procedure; the patient was introduced to the audience 37 years later at the congress of the American Medical Association.

Although general anesthesia started already on "Ether Day" in Boston (16th October 1846), the first successful major abdominal operations including cholecystectomy were performed only at the beginning of 1880s. What had happened during the previous three decades? Surgeons—having now the opportunity to perform painless procedures—had to learn and get experience when to open the abdomen of a living human, where to make the incision, invent tools for these procedures. On 15th July 1882 in Berlin Carl J. A. Langenbuch operated on a 43-year-old man who was suffering from biliary colic for 16 years and became a hopeless morphine addict. Nobody knew the consequences of gallbladder removal. It was the suspicion that lacking a gallbladder would result in continuous bile flow to the intestine resulting in non-treatable diarrhea and, as the consequence of the continuously open sphincter of Oddi, ascending cholangitis could be expected. In the morning following the day of the cholecystectomy Langenbuch entered the room to visit his patient and found him sitting quietly in his bed, smoking a cigar ...

Cholecystectomy as the procedure of choice to solve gallstone disease and its complications was not a glorious march in the end of the nineteenth century. There was no experience for indications: when to operate, in what stage of gallstone disease gallbladder removal should be advised, and anesthesia was also in the developmental stage—the operation itself meant a significant risk factor.

Consequently, cholecystectomy was performed generally at the advanced stage of inflammation, when it was difficult to perform a safe procedure, as a "last chance" to save the patient's life in the hopeless situation. This practice resulted in an extremely high 20% mortality rate during the first few hundred cholecystectomies performed until the dawn of the twentieth century. The majority of surgeons at that time preferred cholecystostomy to gallbladder removal.

That is the main reason why Hans Kehr deserves the recognition, and we can congratulate Professors Berci and Greene for documenting his work and achievements. The German surgeon not only precisely analyzed a large number of cholecystectomies performed by himself but also provided technical advice—including application of his invention, the T-tube, for common bile duct surgery—in his book, published in 1913. This was a considerable help to educate surgeons worldwide also with teaching methods for residents. The wonderful color drawings created by an artist who stood behind Kehr during the procedures and the description of variations in cystic duct and cystic artery anatomy provide additional significance to this book.

It slowly became obvious that *cholecystostomy* cannot offer the final solution to the management of the inflamed stage of cholecystitis—development of a biliary fistula represented a serious event and if the opening of the gallbladder closed spontaneously new gallstones and sometimes malignancies developed in the non-excised organ.

Distinguished surgeons worldwide, like Eugene Polya (inventor of Polya-gastrectomy), suggested at a surgical conference in Budapest in 1908: "It's far better to remove the gallbladder." With the evolution of modern anesthesia, with the development of novel surgical devices and with the expansion of surgical practice the mortality rate of cholecystectomy dropped below 1% worldwide by the 1980s.

Meanwhile, laparoscopy started to conquer medicine. In the beginning, gynecological procedures employed this technology, and later general surgeons on both sides of the Atlantic started to implement laparoscopy. Pioneers H. Kalk in Germany and J. Ruddock in the United States, emphasized the advantage of peritoneoscopy over explorative laparotomy as the diagnostic method for uncertain clinical scenarios. The Veres needle, introduced in 1936, was utilized to create pneumoperitoneum safely.

In the book the authors describe the hard work and achievements of the pioneers of laparoscopic surgery. I have to agree with them: intrigue and enviousness can be observed throughout medical history and this statement is also valid for the evolution of laparoscopic procedures.

When J. Veres published his paper about his invention, the use of the spring-loaded needle—comments were published soon: 1. "have already invented years ago" 2: "have tried it—this needle doesn't work." In 1980, K. Semm, the German gynecologist, performed laparoscopic appendectomy for the first time in medical history. As a consequence, he was sentenced to a brain scan, because "a physician with common sense would not attempt to do this procedure."

When Erich Mühe, the German surgeon who performed the first laparoscopic cholecystectomy in 1985 and a year later reported his method at the congress of German Surgical Society, the audience laughed at him using derogatory remarks like "Mickey Mouse surgery." Phillippe Mouret, a French gynecologist, performed a laparoscopic cholecystectomy in 1987, but he did not have the courage to publish this procedure. His scrub nurse delivered the news of this method to a surgeon in Paris, F. Dubois. He started to perform laparoscopic cholecystectomies and after 18 successful procedures he wanted to publish this new method in the French Medical Journal—but his paper was rejected with the comment: "this is an unacceptable method..."

But the acceptance of laparoscopic cholecystectomy seemed to be unstoppable and the method spread all over the world, like a bush fire. Some referred to this technology as the "perestroika" of surgery.

In 1989, I participated in the World Congress of Surgery in Toronto. One day Prof. Berci advised me to watch a video presentation of a new procedure. This was J. Perissat's presentation of laparoscopic cholecystectomy. It was the first time I have ever seen this new method. I was not convinced at all about the advantages of the laparoscopic approach. What—instead of the classic, safe access, using a long abdominal incision to provide a large, adequate operative field—just pushing 1 cm diameter tubes into the abdominal wall?

Next spring, I received the task at the Annual Congress of the Hungarian Surgical Society to review the nonsurgical treatment options of gallstone disease (litholysis and lithotripsy). At the end of my presentation, I also mentioned that there existed a new surgical method, laparoscopic cholecystectomy. I projected two slides in parallel. One was El Greco's painting of St. Sebastian executed with arrows all over his body. The other slide was a still image of a laparoscopic cholecystectomy. "This (I pointed to the painting) is execution and this (I pointed to the photograph of laparoscopic cholecystectomy) is the new method. No comment!" Thank God, this meeting was also attended by Prof. Berci who thoroughly "washed my brain" and I soon became an enthusiastic laparoscopic surgeon.

It was not easy to convince the surgical community to perform laparoscopic cholecystectomy. Surgical departments went through various stages of acceptance of this method: (1) Non acceptable; (2) Only as an experimental method for animals; (3) Only for specially trained surgeons; (4) I, as the chief of the department, can perform laparoscopic cholecystectomy; (5) All the surgeons at the department apply this method; (6) Conversion is not a shame, this is the right solution in certain cases.

Enthusiastic surgeons in the United States established the Society of American Gastrointestinal and Endoscopic Surgeons (SAGES), which quickly emerged as the most progressive surgical organization with participants from all over the world and took a leading role in the development of safe laparoscopic techniques. Countless educational programs, hands-on training courses, and in-person and virtual conferences are offered for surgeons wishing to specialize in minimally invasive surgery. SAGES organized a comprehensive program, Fundamentals of Laparoscopic Surgery (FLS), which is now a mandatory component of most general surgical residency programs in the United States.

In this book, Drs. Berci and Greene also deal with the present challenges of biliary surgery, like the management of common duct stones and the surgeon's responsibility to apply the safest methods of stone removal. The operative skills we have learned by performing laparoscopic cholecystectomy can be used in further innovative, challenging situations.

During the last three decades new branches of minimally invasive surgery developed: single incision access, natural orifice translumenal endoscopic surgery (NOTES), robotic-assisted surgery, telepresence surgery. We are starting to send astronauts to Mars and other targets in space. Human experiments carried out in special aircrafts producing weightlessness proved that surgical interventions in these circumstances can be performed only in closed systems, like the laparoscopic environment.

When we are learning from the lessons of the pioneer Hans Kehr, we can only concur with Prof. Berci and Prof. Greene, who conclude that this is "An Unfinished Story."

Commentary

Nathaniel J. Soper

During my surgical residency, there was one attending surgeon in private practice who would occasionally perform diagnostic laparoscopy. The residents thought he was crazy for doing these cases, and the junior resident was usually assigned to "assist," that is, watch him. He would glue his eye to the eyepiece of the 0 degree laparoscope and drag his face across the prepped belly while looking at all four quadrants of the abdominal cavity, occasionally inviting the resident to take a peek. I certainly saw no future in this technique or technology…

Fast-forward a few years, and I am now a rookie attending surgeon at Washington University in St. Louis, hired to do maximally invasive surgery and basic science research. Within months of my arrival, Barnes Hospital purchased two (2!) biliary extracorporeal shockwave lithotripsy machines, one controlled by the radiologists and one controlled by a joint effort between G.I. medicine and surgery. We established the Barnes Hospital Gallstone Center to evaluate and treat patients with gallstone disease. The protocol called for an ultrasound to assess the size and number of stones and a CT scan to rule out calcifications in them. Most patients were not candidates for lithotripsy because of stone size, number, or calcifications, and we would then perform a "mini-cholecystectomy" through as small of an incision in the right upper quadrant as possible. The surgeons realized quickly that lithotripsy was not a good solution to gallstone disease—we acknowledged that even when the technique for fragmentation of the stones with subsequent dissolution of the fragments with ursodeoxycholic acid was successful, which was rare, they would almost certainly recur in the future. However, we had established a referral practice for cholecystectomies, and as the junior-most surgeon I was expected to lead the effort for such a mundane disease.

To publicize this "modern approach" to cholelithiasis, I would give outreach educational lectures at rubber chicken dinners around the state. At the end of such a lecture in December of 1988 a nurse asked if I had seen the paper in that month's issue of "Laser Monthly Report" in which Eddie Joe Reddick, MD, was the first to publish the successful outcomes of two patients who had undergone "laparoscopic laser cholecystectomy." The concept to me made eminent sense—take out the diseased gallbladder under direct vision using tiny incisions! Returning to Washington University I was introduced to a urologist who knew of Kurt Semm's work (a gynecologist who had published a case report of a laparoscopic appendectomy) and had contacts at Karl Storz, Inc. Dr. Ralph Clayman and I were able to cobble together rudimentary laparoscopic equipment and performed multiple laparoscopic cholecystectomies in pigs. At that time, it was thought that monopolar cautery used during laparoscopy was dangerous, ergo the use of the laser by Dr. Reddick's group. We did not have a laser, so shrink-wrapped a long cautery probe to 5 mm and demonstrated that this was safe, particularly given the CO_2 environment. The next step for me was to work with our gynecologists to learn how to place laparoscopic ports in humans.

In August of 1989 I called Dr. Reddick's office and was given permission to observe the performance of a laparoscopic laser cholecystectomy at West Side Hospital in Nashville, TN. Five other surgeon observers were in attendance (including Joe Petelin, MD, an early adopter of laparoscopic cholecystectomy). During the first minute of the cholecystectomy performed by Reddick and his partner Doug Olsen it became abundantly clear that this technology represented the future of cholecystectomy, if not of abdominal surgery! The crystal clear and magnified image, the precise dissection, and the easy teamwork made for beautiful and uncomplicated operations. Each of the observers felt the same way and we all left with the plan to start performing these cases as soon as possible.

The only hang-up was that there was no inventory of laparoscopic equipment available for purchase. We ordered a set from Karl Storz, Inc. and were told that we would need to wait to receive it until after it had been exhibited at the Clinical Congress of the American College of Surgeons in Atlanta in October 1989. Two exhibit booths had a looping VHS recording of a laparoscopic laser cholecystectomy done by Reddick's group—the laser company and Karl Storz, Inc. Surgeons were lined up at each of these booths to watch the videotape of the cholecystectomy—at least three-fourths of those surgeons turned away in disgust at such an outlandish procedure whereas one-fourth clamored to purchase the equipment.

Three weeks later—on Friday the 13th of November—we had received the laparoscopic tower and equipment and were ready to try our first clinical case. Because of the novelty of this operation I had decided to include the first 25 patients in an IRB-approved clinical trial, admitting them to our clinical research center and drawing a whole battery of lab tests the following morning. On the day of the operation while I was at the scrub sink preoperatively a senior faculty member warned me that if things did not go well, I would undoubtedly be sued. The female patient had been symptomatic for months while awaiting the operation and had a hydropic gallbladder. The operation was difficult and took four hours to perform, but she did well. Thankfully there were no complications early in our experience and clinical demand exploded. There were several occasions when patients in the preoperative holding area awaiting open cholecystectomy heard about this new technique, cancelled their operations, and scheduled office visits in my clinic.

The next few years were a blur, performing clinical laparoscopic cholecystectomies 3 days per week while teaching others in the institution how to perform these operations. Starting first with the faculty, then chief residents, and ultimately junior residents, all of the general surgeons and trainees had to learn this new technique and technology. Most weekends would be spent teaching at various hands-on courses around the country, including many coordinated by the Society of American Gastrointestinal and Endoscopic Surgeons (SAGES), the only national organization excited to embrace laparoscopic surgery. I remember stating to one of our team members that we should be able to publish several papers about our experience. Unfortunately, the rapid and largely unregulated adoption of this new and radically different technology for performing a common operation led to multiple bile duct injuries over the following decade. Our group articulated and published the concept of dissecting to the "critical view of safety" to minimize the risk of bile duct injury.

Our group was able to quickly establish a laparoscopic surgery research laboratory, the Washington University Institute of Minimally Invasive Surgery, with both technical and financial support from industry. Karl Storz, Inc. supplied the laparoscopic towers and both the US Surgical Corporation and Ethicon supplied disposable trocars and instrumentation. Multiple surgical residents worked in this laboratory over the next decade to help define techniques and refine technology that would facilitate additional laparoscopic operations. Dr. Clayman and his urology fellows also joined our general surgery team to work with industry engineers. They developed a mechanical morcellating device and a bag that would allow safe tissue morcellation within the abdominal cavity. As a result of these collaborative efforts, our team became the first in the world to perform a laparoscopic nephrectomy, just 6 months after our initial cholecystectomy.

Several years went by and I moved on to Northwestern University. Laparoscopic cholecystectomy became the gold standard technique for removing the gallbladder, and it became clear that treatment of common bile duct (CBD) stones discovered at the time of cholecystectomy had essentially disappeared from surgeons' armamentaria. This evolution occurred despite several small prospective trials showing the single stage approach to cholecystectomy and CBD exploration was superior to laparoscopic cholecystectomy with ERCP and stone removal at a second session. Our group at Northwestern, led by Drs. Eric Hungness, B. Fernando Santos, and Ezra Teitelbaum, developed a laparoscopic CBD exploration simulator and established a mastery curriculum that all senior residents were mandated to complete. Critically important, OR nurses from general surgery were then trained, as were the surgeons from the emergency general surgery service. Subsequent studies showed the incidence of laparoscopic CBD exploration to increase significantly at that institution, and that the clinical cost savings were greater than the cost of the simulator and training. This simulation curriculum has subsequently been presented at several academic institutions and at the annual Rural Surgeons hands-on course during the ACS Clinical Congress meeting.

Lessons learned: Not every new technology is of clinical value, and all should initially be viewed with healthy skepticism. When introducing a new clinical technique, great care must be taken to prepare thoroughly for its early performance to minimize harm to patients. Institutional oversight must be in place during such an introduction. Training of established surgeons in new areas of technology is difficult; systems should be developed to facilitate such introduction in a safe fashion. Surgeons performing laparoscopic cholecystectomy still need to understand the dissection principles that will minimize the risk of bile duct injury to their patients. Surgeons performing laparoscopic cholecystectomy should know how to evaluate the CBD intraoperatively and remove CBD stones when they are discovered.

Laparoscopy was truly a revolutionary change in the performance of abdominal surgery; although some patients unfortunately paid a price for this advance, many others have reaped the benefits.

A Personal Glimpse at Bile Duct Injury During Laparoscopic Cholecystectomy

Steven M. Strasberg

In 1989, I was an HPB surgeon at the University of Toronto. I was invited as a consultant to the annual meeting of SAGES, a young society that wanted to increase research output by its membership. At the meeting of the research committee in Louisville, Kentucky, we were engaged in a discussion on whether it would be possible to do a cholecystostomy and stone removal using T-fasteners aided by laparoscopy and fluoroscopy. The meeting was interrupted by a knock on the door. A man was let in, introduced himself, and asked if he could show a video of a laparoscopic cholecystectomy. He had an accent and the chairman of the committee said: "Do you mean a laparoscopic cholecystostomy?" "No." he replied, "I mean a laparoscopic cholecystectomy. I submitted it to the meeting but I missed the deadline and I was told to present it to the research committee." Laparoscopic cholecystectomy? We were in disbelief. Fifteen minutes later, disbelief was replaced with the realization that the surgical world had changed. The man was Jacques Perissat, one of the early French innovators who at that time had done 17 laparoscopic cholecystectomies.

The race was on. This was a major paradigm shift and it was a sudden shift. There have been many advances in laparoscopic surgery since then but they have been incremental. The advent of laparoscopic cholecystectomy was like canoeing over a waterfall, and since then we have been continuing down the river. Laparoscopy was for tubal ligation and most general surgeons had never done it. The instruments were different, the view was different, and you could not touch the tissues. Personally, I was lucky to be on a surgical program with Jacques Perissat twice later that year and by that time his name was well known among general surgeons. With his coaching and a visit to see Charlie McSherry, famous for his publications on cholecystectomy, do his fifth and sixth laparoscopic cholecystectomy in New York City, as well as performing several laparoscopic cholecystectomies in pigs, we were ready to do our first one in Canada. As in many operating rooms, the first time a gallbladder popped out of the small subumbilical incision the room erupted in cheers. After the first 10, we were ready to teach others. But how to train hundreds of surgeons safely? A three-step plan evolved. First, we taught other surgeons in the university. Next, a 2-day course was established to teach community surgeons. The course was run for 2 days, every 2 weeks for 2 years by university surgeons, the first day being laparoscopic cholecystectomy on pigs, and the second, scrubbing as assistants on three laparoscopic cholecystectomies. We asked surgeons to come in pairs so that they would be able to assist each other when establishing the procedure in their hospital. Finally, university surgeons traveled out to community hospitals as coaches when the procedure was being established. We were also coached by visitors such as Barry Mckernan from Georgia, who came to Toronto and encouraged us to be two-handed laparoscopic surgeons.

In a landmark paper, the first large-scale report on the results of laparoscopic cholecystectomy in North America was published in the *New England Journal of Medicine* in April of 1991 [20]. Five thousand eighteen patients had been treated in multiple institutions in the south of the United States with a conversion rate of under 5%. But ominously this paper, whose lead author was by William Meyers of Duke University, reported that the bile duct injury rate was 0.5%, about five times higher than reported rates for open cholecystectomy. This was unexpected. It seemed that the bile duct injury rate dropped to normal after the first 13 procedures. However, soon other reports also indicated that biliary injury was definitely and highly increased in laparoscopic cholecystectomy. Soon after, the most common mechanism of major injury, the so-called classic injury, was described again by surgeons at Duke University [21]. By late 1992, all of this was consolidated in an NIH consensus conference on laparoscopic cholecystectomy which concluded that the benefits of laparoscopic cholecystectomy exceeded its risks, recognizing that bile duct injury was an ongoing problem. The proceedings of this conference were published in a single issue of the *American Journal of Surgery* in April 1993. For those interested in the history of laparoscopic cholecystectomy, the more than 160 pages of this issue of the journal have become a historical goldmine.

After arriving at Washington University in Saint Louis in 1992, I received a steady stream of patients with bile duct injuries of various types. In 1995, in an analytical review written with Martin Hertl and Nathaniel Soper, we described a new classification of biliary injuries which took into account injuries which seem to be occurring more frequently in the laparoscopic era [22]. Parts of it were based on Henri Bismuth's classification of benign biliary strictures. Also, it was clear from the "classic injury" paper that misidentification was a key factor in major injuries. So, in the same article we described a method of ductal identification whose goal was to avoid misidentification. The new Critical View of Safety Method was based on a method of ductal identification in open cholecystectomy in which the cystic duct and artery were putatively identified but not finally identified until the gallbladder was completely freed from the liver and was hanging by these two structures only [22]. When we tried taking the whole gallbladder off the cystic plate laparoscopically in this way, we found it made clipping of the cystic structure somewhat awkward and by the time the method was introduced only the lower one-third of the gallbladder was required to be removed from the cystic plate.

With the description of this method, we naively thought that the incidence of biliary injuries would drop considerably. But 5 years later, by reading operative notes of biliary injuries we realized that misidentification was alive and well by virtue of the continued use of the infundibular view method of ductal identification. This method, which depends on identification of the funnel shaped junction of the cystic duct with the lower end of the gallbladder, was identified as being unreliable in the face of severe inflammation because, with retractile inflammation of the hepatocystic triangle, the junction of the common bile duct with the inflammatory mass takes on a deceptive funnel-shape [23].

Hans Kehr, the subject of this book, was the first surgeon to describe subtotal cholecystectomy as a bailout procedure in badly inflamed gallbladders in 1898. Bile duct injuries are much more common in the face of severe inflammation, both acute and chronic, as shown convincingly in studies by Bjorn Tornqvist [24] REF and Ewen Griffiths [25] and their colleagues. One hundred twenty years after Kehr first described the operation, subtotal fenestrating cholecystectomy is becoming the bailout procedure of choice when local conditions do not allow achievement of the Critical View of Safety [26].

The recently published Consensus Conference on Safe Cholecystectomy led by Michael Brunt of Washington University was focused on avoidance of bile duct injury and is required reading for those interested in the subject. A glimpse of the future can be seen in recent reports of the potential role for artificial intelligence in cholecystectomy [27]. I feel certain that in the future, robots will become adept at anatomic identification, possibly a step on the way to autorobotic surgery.

This has been a brief subjective overview of a complex subject.

My "Rebirth" as a "Laparoscopic" Surgeon: And What that Means for Surgeons Today

Lee Swanstrőm

I finished my surgical residency in 1988. I had a year to kill before my Fellowship in surgical endoscopy at University of Western Ontario started, so I was looking for opportunities. I had been invited to join a premier surgical practice at our community based tertiary care hospital. I had taken this position because this group was the largest tertiary referral for complex foregut pathologies in the state—and this was my main interest. They strongly urged me to obtain further training in flexible endoscopy which is what led me to apply to one of the few institutions that would train surgeons in advanced procedures like ERCP. Unfortunately, I was only accepted for the following year so, as I said, I had a year to kill. Having done part of my undergraduate training in France, and speaking French, I had subscribed to some French surgical newsletters in order to practice my French. These newsletters were filled with controversy in the summer of 1988 over the presentations of Messieurs Mouret, Perrisat, and Dubois on a new procedure: "Cholécystectomie par celioscopie." These reports were mostly negative, even condescending, and therefore, were all the more interesting to me. Anyway, to make a long story short, I ended up traveling to Paris in early 1989, watching François Dubois perform these cases in his lab(!) and then traveling to Tutlingen, Germany, by train to buy in person, a set of Storz GYN laparoscopy instruments—as instrument orders by traditional channels were already 2 years in backorder as a result of the gold rush to this new procedure. Amazing to think that in this era, the biggest bottleneck to adoption of a radical new procedure was not federal regulations, was not reimbursement issues, was not documentation of training or competence—it was purely that there were not enough laparoscopic tools to satisfy the demand. The instruments I bought (cash!) were in a special suitcase, black with foam cutouts for each instrument. Traveling back to the United States, I kept it with me and it traveled in the overhead bin on the plane—if you can imagine today!

This story is certainly not unique, there was a generation of us at the time, old and young, who scrambled to learn "Lap chole." For me and many others, it was not so much a desire to learn laparoscopy, or to do a better (safer? cheaper?) cholecystectomy, it was the excitement of a paradigm shift in how we treated patients. The concept of not damaging or hurting a patient in pursuit of their surgical cure was as alien as it was exciting for those of us looking for a radical change in the surgical world. It was pivotal in the sense that it empowered patients and put their concerns at the forefront of treatment decisions and the future evolution of surgery—both procedure wise and for technology development. I believe the fact that it was cholecystectomy initiating this particular pivotal moment in the history of surgery was important. Because the procedure was so common, and so well defined—at least since the time of Hans Kehr—led to a frustrated desire to make it better (e.g., electro-shock wave lithotripsy (ESWL), ursodiol, mini-lap chole) but it also created an opportunity to force an attitude shift in the whole of general surgery. Performing cholecystectomies was an absolute necessity for a general surgeon of the day. If a better way happened, and patients demanded it, all surgeons had to adopt it—or retire. I am convinced that if it would have been another disruptive minimally invasive treatment that happened, such as trans-arterial valve replacement (TAVR) for example, the impact would not have been as systemic. This is perhaps simply because the case numbers are fewer and the majority of surgeons could have sneaked by without learning, letting others shoulder the risk of a new procedure and do it, without impacting their practices.

So, lap chole represented a seismic shift in the way surgery was thought of world wide. After the tumultuous decade of lap chole introduction that followed, where there was a mad stampede of general surgeons to learn laparoscopy, where "new" surgical societies (SAGES) rose in prominence and where industry re-tooled to make a new generation of instrumentation, "minimally invasive" became an almost mandatory adjective to describe any new surgical approach, or one's practice specialty, or how we approached patients when discussing surgery [28]. Likewise, industry made this their new benchmark for product development—if it was not less invasive, there was no interest [29]. This all took place way before the consideration of "evidence based" practice, and it was decades before there was first degree evidence supporting laparoscopic over open cholecystectomy, and even with early and persisting reports of common duct injuries being widely available patients uniformly refused to accept an open cholecystectomy over a minimally invasive alternative [30].

I said that it was not so much the laparoscopy that was the significant change, but the concern for the patient impact. This was made apparent when 10 years after the laparoscopic tsunami, a proposal for an even less invasive approach compared to laparoscopy was advocated, by many of us who had in fact participated in the dawn of lap chole. This of course was the natural orifice translumenal surgery (NOTES) phenomenon, a concept advocating totally incisionless and potentially pain free surgery by using flexible endoscopy and natural orifice access [31] Once again cholecystectomy was picked as a target, possibly because the originators of the concept were hoping to once again force a generational paradigm shift as had happened in laparoscopy. Perhaps this was in fact a little too intentional and forced, as in the end it never really panned out. I think surgeons at the time, nervously watched for the reactions of their patient to this concept and thus created a demand for more evidence, and when it turned out that patients were rather blasé, the surgical community, exhausted by more than a decade of disruption, endless reeducation, learning curves, etc., breathed a sigh of relief and went about their minimally invasive business as normal [32]. There was also the fact that industry was newly restrained by the FDA and other regulatory agencies from giving surgeons access to "weapons of mass destruction" without thorough vetting and training to prevent the bad outcomes seen in the early days of lap chole. Finally, there was also the fact that NOTES was technically many times more difficult to learn and almost impossible to practice as safely as even laparoscopic cholecystectomy [33]. Anyway, NOTES did not happen for cholecystectomy, though it subsequently has happened for other procedures like rectal resection and achalasia treatments [34].

So, today we are still waiting for the next great paradigm shift in surgical patient care. It is hard to say if it will again focus on cholecystectomy or not, though it remains a good candidate as it is moderately complex, mildly dangerous to patients, very common and therefore a critical component of most surgeon's practices. What it will look like is hard to say, maybe robotics, although the current state of robotic laparoscopic cholecystectomy probably does not qualify, as it is really only about the surgeon and not about the patient. Maybe Artificial Intelligence (AI) in surgical decision making? Maybe augmented imaging? Maybe realization of the dream of George Berci and others to eliminate common duct injuries. Maybe even the old NOTES dream of incisionless surgery. Wouldn't that be exciting?

Technology Advance in Surgery in Both Worlds: Long-Term Personal Overview

Tehemton Erach Udwadia

Since the dawn of surgery there have been only three really genuine patient-friendly Revolutions: Anesthesia which relieved the patient of the physical, emotional, and mental torture of pain and suffering during surgery, Asepsis which has greatly reduced the high morbidity and mortality of postoperative infection, Minimal Access Surgery which has reduced pain, hospitalization, cost, medication, scarring, and most important permitted early return to home, family, work.

In 1972, my Ward at the J.J. Hospital Bombay, a Charity Teaching Hospital, with an allotted bed strength of 20 patients, had at any one time, 50 to 70 patients in the Ward, on the beds, on mattresses between beds, under the beds, in the corridor all the way to the washroom, in the main corridor all the way to the elevator. Having a tertiary care GI and HPB Unit in addition to a General Surgery Unit, the backlog was heavy because of constant referrals. The overburdened infrastructure had just no investigative facilities available, hence the backlog. When I saw a gynecologist colleague do a laparoscopy, I realized that laparoscopy was the answer to improve both investigation and bed turnover. The laparoscope was brought in 1972 for surgical use for the first time in India and the developing world, not as a tribute to technology advance, but merely as a diagnostic tool to help early diagnosis in an impoverished Teaching Hospital for the poor. In addition to visual diagnosis, it provided a guided biopsy diagnosis. Few years later, a paper was presented on Early Experience of Diagnostic Laparoscopy in Surgery at the First International Conference on Tropical Surgery in Mumbai. At the end of the presentation, the Chairman declared that he was not a coward, he entered the abdomen through wide open doors, not like this sissy who peeps through the keyholes of my doors, to the laughter and applause of the audience. That was a bugle call to action.

I researched the literature and found confidence that two other surgeons, George Berci and Alfred Cuschieri were committed to the value of Diagnostic Laparoscopy. I found surgeons in small towns and rural areas were far more receptive. They often lacked x-rays but thanks to the strong family planning program in India in the mid-1970s, some already had laparoscopes. They just had to reverse the table tilt and look toward the diaphragm and they were in a better position for early diagnosis than their city colleagues. Traveling extensively over small town and rural India to promote diagnostic laparoscopy, I was humbled to see the qualities of strength, character, innovation, improvisation, and total dedication of the small-town surgeon in India who at personal sacrifice were giving relief to over 70% of the country's population [35]. This travel also helped make friends and prepare fertile ground for the laparoscopic cholecystectomy avalanche that was to follow.

When the first laparoscopic cholecystectomy was done in the developing world in 1990 by the Surgical Team of Ward 19A, J. J. Hospital, we were immediately drowned in criticism. British surgeons wrote in Indian Journals that sophisticated surgery was inappropriate and had no place in the developing world [36]. Indian Surgeons wrote in British Journals questioning our ethics, morality, and suggesting that we were stooges of the West [37]. I replied that the poor had as much right to less expense, less pain, and short hospital stay with the great economic benefit to daily wages manual laborers of the developing world of early return to work and earning. MAS had its ultimate advantage and benefit for and in the developing world.

Technology advance in High Income Countries is growing at an incredible pace, altering the practice of surgery. This may have its downside in patient care. In time, if not now, it could happen that a Laparoscopic Surgeon may be forced, to ensure safety, by converting to open cholecystectomy. To do a nasty open cholecystectomy with no prior experience of open cholecystectomy could necessitate the urgent services of a Hepato-Biliary Surgeon.

When we discuss the Introduction of New Technology into developing countries there are two surgeries in developing countries: the surgery done in large five star hospitals in the cities which can be comparable to the best in the world and surgery done in small town and rural areas. In this second level of surgery, the Introduction of Technology is greatly facilitated by one often unrecognized factor. The steel of the small town and rural surgeon has been forged in the furnace of deprivation, necessity, want, and has matured with ingenuity, innovation, and a determination to do better. Further they have a bond with their patients which ensure a certain degree of safety. This surgeon can adapt to any technology if given the opportunity because this surgeon is a master in the ultimate super-specialty—General Surgery. They can trephine for an extradural bleed, do a Caesarean section for obstructed labor, and manage a polytrauma. The opportunity they need for the introduction of new technology has only two aspects, cost and training.

Cost: Every piece of equipment used in the pursuit of new technology in a developing country MUST be REUSABLE. The major cost of Minimal Access Surgery is the optics. One can only operate on what one sees. The cost of the camera and the telescope is often reduced by like-minded surgeons forming a group to purchase one set. All the other equipment, light source, insufflator, and all hand instruments are locally manufactured in most developing countries with acceptable quality and affordable cost. As important as initial cost is instrument care, which is always far better when the surgeon has paid for the equipment, than when the hospital has. One set of diagnostic laparoscopy equipment can last over 18 years for over 3000 patients [38]. Equally important for cost containment for the patient is to ensure complication—free surgery. Every complication adds to the cost of surgery.

Training: Simple training equipment, very often self-made, can be just as effective as virtual reality and state of the Art Training Center. Training requires patience, persistence, precision, and practice. Practice does not make perfect; precise perfect practice makes perfect. National minimal access surgery associations like the Indian Association of Gastrointestinal Endo-Surgeons (IAGES) can play a great role in introducing MAS, imparting sustained training courses, credentialing, proctoring, and ensuring cost containment as seen in countries like Brazil or India. Safety is equally an issue in every country, worldwide. Safety is not only technologically driven; it is surgeon dependent. An essential part of training and mentorship is to make the trainees aware of their limitations, never to exceed them and to put the devil of hubris behind them. In small towns and rural areas, the patient is not a number on the operation list, and every patient is a part of the surgeon's extended family. Safety is intuitive and imperative. IAGES holds courses in small towns all over the country in basic laparoscopic surgery as also in specific procedures like hernia. Distance learning and mentoring are playing a progressive role in maintaining vigil on standards of proficiency, safety, and basic training in developing countries.

The only truth in surgery is change. New technology for surgical advance will always flow; much will replace the old. We are at a time when each surgeon must view new technology pragmatically and dispassionately without succumbing to hype, or jumping on the bandwagon. Every surgeon must decide if new surgical technology is not true surgical progress, is more for the benefit of the manufacturer, or is this technology truly real surgical progress for the surgeon and the patient. I for one would never permit my gallbladder to be removed through a rent in my rectum, nor with the use of a robot. I have for decades maintained that for technology to be applicable to the developing world it must confirm to the five A test: Affordable, Available, Accessible, Acceptable, and Appropriate.

We believe that surgeons are an international community. How many of us really do look beyond our own hospital, city, country? We look forward to mini-robots measuring nanometers, smaller than an atom, as new technology. Were we to study the Lancet Commission on Global Surgery [39], we would realize that aid available for repair of a strangulated hernia, for a Caesarian section for obstructed labor, or for a compound fracture would be new technology for five billion people who have little access to safe, affordable, and available surgery.

Reflections of a Trainee During the Laparoscopic Cholecystectomy Revolution 1989–1992

Sherry M. Wren

1989—I will never forget the initial reaction to laparoscopic cholecystectomy by the senior academic surgeons at Yale. I was a third-year resident and listened intently to attendings debating the lack of merit of this new approach with comments such as "I would not do that to my dog," "it's malpractice," and "what is wrong with the mini-cholecystectomies we are already doing—that's less invasive surgery." These comments were said with an authority and a finality that did not encourage open discussion. Shortly, there was a change in attitude and interest as three things happened. First, private practice surgeons in the community rapidly adopted and marketed the new technique; second, junior attendings saw an opportunity and wanted to innovate and change practice; and third, patients increasingly desired this new procedure and there was a need to stay competitive in the marketplace. With a change of heart senior surgeons then decided to learn the procedure. I remember watching the initial cases and later realized I saw the first surgical revolution of my career. It was exciting, I did not pause to think that weekend courses on pigs may not be a great training paradigm and how patients were basically providing the real learning platform for this revolution and that they had to pay the price for this haphazard education model.

I left clinical residency training for my research time and returned to a changed world as a PGY 4 in 1992. Attending surgeons were still "learners," and laparoscopic cholecystectomy had irreversibly changed the landscape of surgery forever. The number of cholecystectomies being performed in the United States had inexplicably and exponentially increased. In Connecticut there was an increase of 29% of cholecystectomies being performed laparoscopically between 1990 and 1991 [40]. Nationwide, by 1992 there was an astounding near doubling of the rate of cholecystectomy in claims data from 1.35 per 1000 enrollees in 1988 to 2.15 in 1992 [41]. There was significant speculation as to the reasons for this increase in volume but no definitive data was ever published. With this increase in volume there were now reports of new and unheard-of complications such as major vascular injury, intestinal injuries from laparoscopic access, as well as significant increases in bile duct injury (BDI). In 1989 the overall mortality for open cholecystectomy was 0.17% with a BDI rate of 0.2% [42]. By 1992, there was a reported incidence of 0.59% BDI, 0.25% vascular injury, and 0.14% intestinal injuries [43]. Even though Dr. Berci described intraoperative fluorocholangiography in 1978 this was not commonly being taught or practiced [44]. Despite data showing IOC could lower the risk of BDI, only 21.5% of surgeons reported performing routine intraoperative cholangiogram (IOC) in >75% of their laparoscopic cholecystectomies [45]. I left residency in 1994 believing that I had been well trained in the performance of laparoscopic cholecystectomy. At that time, I had never done an IOC, soon this was about to change after moving to Los Angeles to start a hepatobiliary (HPB) fellowship.

LA County USC Medical Center is located in East Los Angeles with a primarily Hispanic local community population resulting in an incredible volume of gallbladder disease. Patients often waited significant amounts of time and had multiple episodes of cholecystitis before undergoing surgery and therefore often had "difficult gallbladders." Six months into my fellowship I discharged a patient after a routine cholecystectomy and later had to readmit him with bile peritonitis due to my first and only BDI. I was horrified to discover he did not have a cystic duct leak but the classic injury pattern of excision of a piece of common bile duct, clipped distal duct, and fortunately no vascular injury. I reoperated and repaired the injury with a hepaticojejunostomy and the patient recovered without any further sequelae. I could not understand how I injured the duct and replayed the operation endlessly through my head which offered no insight into how I could have made such a serious error. I was not aware at the time of the work by Way et al. demonstrating that this is often an error of misperception as opposed to skill, knowledge, or judgment [46]. Fortunately, at this time I was introduced to Dr. George Berci who was visiting from across town in Los Angeles. Dr. Berci was passionate about safe cholecystectomy technique and I began to understand the procedure in a way I had not previously and soon became a routine cholangiographer for all cases. I never wanted to repeat the error I had made and realized that a properly done IOC added a degree of safety to what was dismissed as a routine, simple operation. When I completed fellowship and joined the faculty in 1995 this chance meeting with a cross-town expert had set the stage for a longstanding relationship with Dr. Berci and dedication to improving the safety of cholecystectomy through teaching fluorocholangiography, laparoscopic common bile duct operations, and always searching for opportunities for procedure and safety improvement.

An additional invaluable lesson from those years spent as a trainee during the MIS revolution was how innovation and technology advances will occur in your surgical career and you must evaluate each advance and decide whether to embrace the change or not. Seeing first-hand what happened to surgeons who refused to learn laparoscopy and then were quickly left behind and obsolete, left an indelible impression on me. As faculty, I advanced my practice in minimally invasive surgery as an early adopter for other GI conditions and fully adopted laparoscopy for intestinal cancer resections from 1997 onwards. Soon more disruptive technologies were being innovated and by 2005 it was obvious that surgical robotics and natural orifice translumenal endoluminal surgery (NOTES) were innovations I needed to evaluate and decide whether I was going to acquire. The time and effort necessary to learn a new operative technique or platform should not be underestimated; there is a significant amount of preparation, reading, practice, and slower OR times as you learn and practice the new technique. The specter of the informal education process and unregulated wide adoption of laparoscopic cholecystectomy colored my future procedural adoption and expectations for education about the new techniques. After much consideration I decided that robotics was going to be the area of investment of my time and effort and I would not embark on a learning journey with NOTES. At the time I worried whether I was making the correct decision. There was a lot of press and I did not want to be like the recalcitrant surgeons who spurned laparoscopy. Fortunately, my decision to choose robotics was the correct one and has brought significant professional growth. The current organized robotic educational training program with simulators, online education modules, and dry and wet labs demonstrates the incredible journey from laparoscopic cholecystectomy training in 1989 via weekend courses prior to doing a first case. Education is now firmly embedded in many new technologies from robotics to endovascular procedures primarily because of the legacy of the haphazard training for laparoscopic cholecystectomy. Fortunately, surgeons and surgical societies learned the lessons from those early days of laparoscopic cholecystectomy wherein a dramatic change in the practice of surgery occurs but with no organized means by which to adopt, teach, and evaluate the technological advance. Laparoscopic cholecystectomy remains the best example of what can happen when a technological advance causes a seismic shift in how things are done and the myriad positive and negative ripple effects downstream. We continue to reflect and learn from this experience and try to not repeat many of the mistakes unknowingly made during that time.

References

Commentary: Berci-Greene "No Stones Left Unturned" Kehr Book

1. Reynolds W, Jr. The first laparoscopic cholecystectomy. JSLS 2001;5:89–94.
2. Morgenstern L. An unsung hero of the laparoscopic revolution: Eddie Joe Reddick. Surg Innov 2008; 15: 245–248.
3. Brunt LM. SAGES presidential address: A SAGES Magical Mystery Tour. Surg Endosc 2015; 29:3423–3431.
4. George Berci: Trials, Triumphs, Innovations. A SAGES & Cine-Med Production, 2013.
5. Pucher PH, Brunt LM, Fanelli RD, Asbun HJ, Aggarwal R (2015) SAGES expert Delphi consensus: critical factors for safe surgical practice in laparoscopic cholecystectomy. Surg Endosc 29:3074–3085. https://doi.org/10.1007/s00464-015-4079-z
6. https://www.sages.org/safe-cholecystectomy-program/
7. Brunt LM, Deziel DJ, Telem DA, et al. Safe cholecystectomy multi-society practice guideline and state of the art consensus conference on prevention of bile duct Injury during cholecystectomy. Ann Surg 2020; 272:3–23 and Surg Endosc 2020; 34:2827–2855.
8. Strasberg SM, Hertl M, Soper NJ. An analysis of the problem of biliary injury during laparoscopic cholecystectomy. J Am Coll Surg 1995; 180:101–125

The Trajectory of Biliary Surgery: Personal Reflections

9. Deziel DJ. The Journey of the Surgeon-Hero. Surg Endosc (2008) 22:1–7.
10. McSherry CK and the EDAP Investigators Group. The Results of the EDAP Multicenter Trial of Biliary Lithotripsy in the United States. Surg Gynecol Obstet (1991) 173: 461–464.
11. Deziel DJ, Millikan KW, Economou SG, et al. Complications of Laparoscopic Cholecystectomy: A National Survey of 4,292 Hospitals and Analysis of 77,604 Cases. Am J Surg (1993) 165: 9–14.
12. Brunt LM, Deziel DJ, Telem DA, et al. Safe Cholecystectomy Multi-society Practice Guideline and State of the Art Consensus Conference on Prevention of Bile Duct Injury During Cholecystectomy. Ann Surg (2020) 272: 3–23.
13. Brunt LM, Deziel DJ, Telem DA, et al. Safe Cholecystectomy Multi-society Practice Guideline and State of the Art Consensus Conference on Prevention of Bile Duct Injury During Cholecystectomy. Surg Endosc (2020) 34: 2827-2855.
14. Cortez AR, Potts III JR. More of Less: General Surgery Resident Experience in Biliary Surgery. J Am Coll Surg (2020) 231: 33–42.
15. Deziel DJ, Veenstra BR. Biliary anatomy. In: The SAGES Manual of Biliary Surgery. Asbun H, Shah MM, Ceppa E, Auyang E, editors. Springer, NY, NY, 2020. ISBN 978-3-030-13275-0.
16. Moore FD. Metabolic Care of the Surgical Patient. WB Saunders Co. Philadelphia, 1959.

Laparoscopic Cholecystectomy: At the Beginning…1989–1990

17. Hunter JG. Avoidance of bile duct injury during laparoscopic cholecystectomy. Am J Surg 1991; 162:71–76.

Personal Perspective/Experience—In This Surgical Space

18. Traverso LW, K Kozarek RA. In Bile Ducts & Bile Duct Stones. G.Berci and A. Cuschieri, eds. WB Saunders, Philadelphia. 1997, pp. 154–160.
19. Perissat J, Huibregtse, K, Keane FBV, et al Management of bile duct stones in the era of laparoscopic cholecystectomy. British J Surg, 1994; 81:799–810.

A Personal Glimpse at Bile Duct Injury During Laparoscopic Cholecystectomy

20. Southern Surgical Club. A prospective analysis of 1518 laparoscopic cholecystectomies. New Engl J of Med. 324:1073–8, 1991.
21. Davidoff AM; Pappas TN; Murray EA; Hilleren DJ; Johnson RD; Baker ME; Newman GE; Cotton PB; Meyers WC. Mechanisms of major biliary injury during laparoscopic cholecystectomy. Mechanisms of major biliary injury during laparoscopic cholecystectomy. Ann Surg. 215:196–202, 1992.
22. Strasberg SM; Hertl M; Soper JN: An analysis of the problem of biliary injury during laparoscopic cholecystectomy. J Am Coll Surg 180:101–25, 1995.
23. Strasberg SM; Eagon CJ; Drebin JA: The "Hidden Cystic Duct" Syndrome and the Infundibular Technique of Laparoscopic Cholecystectomy – the Danger of the False Infundibulum. J Am Coll of Surg, 191:661–7, 2000.
24. Tornqvist B; Waage A; Zheng Z; Ye W; Nilsson M. Severity of Acute Cholecystitis and Risk of Iatrogenic Bile Duct Injury During Cholecystectomy, a Population-Based Case-Control Study. World J Surg. 40:1060–7, 2016.

25. Griffiths EA; Hodson J; Vohra RS; Marriott P; Katbeh T; Zino S; Nassar AHM; West Midlands Research Collaborative. Utilisation of an operative difficulty grading scale for laparoscopic cholecystectomy. Surg Endosc. 33(1):110–121, 2019.
26. Strasberg SM; Pucci MJ; Brunt LM; Deziel DJ. Subtotal Cholecystectomy "Fenestrating" vs "Reconstituting" Subtypes and the Prevention of Bile Duct Injury: Definition of the Optimal Procedure in Difficult Operative Conditions. J Am Coll Surg. 222:89–96, 2016.
27. Mascagni P; Vardazaryan A; Alapatt D; Urade T; Emre T; Fiorillo C; Pessaux P; Mutter D; Marescaux J; Costamagna G; Dallemagne B; Padoy N Artificial Intelligence for Surgical Safety: Automatic Assessment of the Critical View of Safety in Laparoscopic Cholecystectomy Using Deep Learning. Ann Surg Nov 16, 2020.

My "Rebirth" as a "Laparoscopic" Surgeon: And What that Means for Surgeons Today

28. Spaner SJ, Warnock GL. A Brief History of Endoscopy, Laparoscopy, and Laparoscopic Surgery. Journal of Laparoendoscopic & Advanced Surgical Techniques, Vol. 7, No. 6. Published Online:30 Jan 2009. https://doi.org/10.1089/lap.1997.7.369
29. A Bhidé, Bowler CN, Datar S. Case Histories of Significant Medical Advances: Laparoscopy. Harvard Business School Case Studies Series https://www.hbs.edu/faculty/Publication%20Files/20-008_cfca0c4d-a132-4d00-a299-c28f2a93ac3d.pdf
30. Archer SB, Brown DB, Smith CD, Branum GD, Hunter JG. Bile Duct Injury During Laparoscopic Cholecystectomy: Results of a National Survey. Ann Surg. 2001 Oct; 234(4): 549–559.
31. Giday SA, Kantsevoy SV, Kalloo AN. Principle and history of Natural Orifice Transluminal Endoscopic Surgery (NOTES), Minimally Invasive Therapy & Allied Technologies, (2006) 15:6, 373–377, https://doi.org/10.1080/13645700601038010
32. Volkman ET, Hungness ES, Soper NJ, Swanström LL. "Surgeon Perceptions of Natural Orifice Transluminal Endoscopic Surgery (NOTES)." J Gastrointestinal Surg. 2009 Aug;13(8):1401–10.
33. Potter K, Swanström LL. Potter K, Swanström LL. "Natural orifice surgery (NOTES) and biliary disease, is there a role?" Journal of Hepato-Biliary-Pancreatic Surgery. 0944-1166 (Print) 1436-0691 Volume 16, Number 3 / May, 2009
34. Spaun, G., Swanström, L. Quo vadis NOTES?. Eur Surg 40, 211–219 (2008). https://doi.org/10.1007/s10353-008-0428-7.

Technology Advance in Surgery in Both Worlds: Long-Term Personal Overview

35. Udwadia T.E (2003) Surgical Care for the Poor. A personal Indian Perspective. Indian J. Surgery 65:504–509
36. Chesylin-Curtis S (1991) Laparoscopic Cholecystectomy. National Med J India 4:155–156
37. Antia N.H (1994) Key Hole Surgery. Lancet 344:396–397
38. Maryam Alfa-Wali, Samuel Osaghae (2017) Practise, Future, Training and Safety of laparoscopy in LMIC. World Journal of Gastrointestinal Surgery 9:13–18
39. Lancet Commission on Rural Surgery (2015)

Reflections of a Trainee During the Laparoscopic Cholecystectomy Revolution 1989–1992

40. Orlando R, Russell JC, Lynch J, Mattie A. Laparoscopic Cholecystectomy: A Statewide Experience. Arch Surg. 1993;128(5):494–499. https://doi.org/10.1001/archsurg.1993.01420170024002
41. Legorreta AP, Silber JH, Costantino GN, Kobylinski RW, Zatz SL. Increased Cholecystectomy Rate After the Introduction of Laparoscopic Cholecystectomy. JAMA. 1993;270(12):1429–1432.
42. Roslyn JJ, Binns GS, Hughes EF, Saunders-Kirkwood K, Zinner MJ, Cates JA. Open cholecystectomy. A contemporary analysis of 42,474 patients. Ann Surg. 1993;218(2):129–137. https://doi.org/10.1097/00000658-199308000-00003.
43. Deziel DJ, Millikan KW, Economou SG, Doulas A, Ko ST, Airan MC. Complications of laparoscopic cholecystectomy: a national survey of 4,292 hospitals and an analysis of 77,604 cases. Am J Surg. 1993;165(1):9–14. https://doi.org/10.1016/s0002-9610(05)80397-6
44. Berci G, Shore JM, Hamlin JA, Morgenstern L. Operative fluoroscopy and cholangiography. The use of modern radiologic technics during surgery. Am J Surg. 1978;135(1):32–35. https://doi.org/10.1016/0002-9610(78)90005-3
45. Flum DR, Dellinger EP, Cheadle A, Chan L, Koepsell T. Intraoperative Cholangiography and Risk of Common Bile Duct Injury During Cholecystectomy. JAMA. 2003;289(13):1639–1644. https://doi.org/10.1001/jama.289.13.1639
46. Way LW, Stewart L, Gantert W, et al. Causes and prevention of laparoscopic bile duct injuries: analysis of 252 cases from a human factors and cognitive psychology perspective. Ann Surg. 2003;237(4):460–469. https://doi.org/10.1097/01.SLA.0000060680.92690.E9

Part IV
Looking to the Future

Epilogue

Recommendations for the Future of Surgical Treatment of Biliary Stone Disease

> Disease is very old and nothing about it has changed. It is we who change as we learn what was formerly imperceptible. –Charcot

There were several reasons to begin this monograph with a translation of Dr. Kehr's book on biliary surgery: (a) he recommended over a century ago the importance of training surgeons; (b) he espoused the importance of teaching anatomy and displaying the arterial and biliary systems in color; (c) he advocated the diagnosis and removal of common duct stones during the same operative session.

Three decades ago, the introduction of laparoscopic cholecystectomy (LC) opened a new chapter in biliary surgery. What did we learn during the past three decades regarding laparoscopic surgery and the management of bile duct stones? We should have learned that the basic principles espoused by Hans Kehr have not really changed in the transition from an open to a minimally invasive approach for gallbladder removal and clearance of stones from the extrahepatic bile ducts. The disruptive introduction of new technology forced all surgeons who performed cholecystectomy and traditional approaches to choledocholithiasis to either embrace laparoscopic approaches or risk being excluded from taking care of a significant portion of their patient base. The financial implications of eschewing this new technology would be potentially enormous. The fear of working through long instruments inside the abdomen rather than having hands proximate to the operative anatomy was potentially daunting. The approaches to teaching this new technology to both mature surgeons and surgical trainees were intimidating to the most seasoned academic attending surgeon. Despite all of this, the introduction of laparoscopic cholecystectomy could not be assuaged because patients demanded it.

Training Courses

The laparoscopic approach required a completely new surgical training paradigm and way of thinking. Traditional academic teaching programs were slow to embrace the importance of this new technique. Most professional surgical societies were equally languid in assuming leadership especially in controlling the introduction of this new way of operating. Only a few surgeons in the private sector embraced the technology and saw the potential of this new operative approach. These surgeons began to work with the small group of instrument and scope manufacturers who also realized the potential market. The overall concept was that promulgation of laparoscopic surgery could not be controlled through traditional training or the application of clinical trials to assess safety and efficacy. The horse was out of the barn!

Thankfully, one very young, but visionary, surgical organization, SAGES, created well-designed teaching courses that were offered in various cities during the weekend to allow practicing surgeons to at least gain technical familiarity through operating on animal models. These courses were supported by instrument companies and featured mentoring surgeons who had become familiar with these techniques only recently at their home institutions. Certifications were generated to document these weekend experiences so that individual surgeons could have something to satisfy the primitive credentialing and privileging guidelines at their own hospitals. Of course, the number of surgeons requiring courses far exceeded the few, well-developed opportunities for training that were available. Following these hands-on experiences and despite recommendations for laparoscopic surgical neophytes to work with a monitor at their own institution, many decided to immediately transition to operating upon waiting patients.

Consequently, over the next few years the complications resulting from laparoscopic cholecystectomy including bile duct injury (BDI) increased significantly and were associated with mortality. SAGES produced information, policies, guidelines, and instructions to improve the existing conditions. SAGES also initiated a number of educational courses, publications, and a multi-institutional report to describe the various areas of analysis and improvements. It was recognized early in the laparoscopic revolution that procedures and resultant complications were being underreported due to a lack of well-structured outcomes registries. As compared with the experience in the United States, other countries (e.g., Sweden) with a centralized recording system were able to report more accurate data. The major issue was that we did not insist or create in a timely fashion a national recording system to track operative results. This issue was ameliorated as newer operations involving laparoscopic approaches were introduced.

Intraoperative Cholangiography, Anatomy, Bile Leakage, and Stone Identification

The introduction of well-performed intraoperative cholangiography (IOC) was crucial to display the anatomy at the initial operation and to demonstrate anatomical anomalies or ductal injury that would benefit from immediate repair. The hard lesson, however, was that many surgeons who recognized ductal injuries were not skilled enough to repair them. Delayed realization of injuries, especially without performance of IOC, became common and required patients to be transferred to academic biliary services for ultimate repair. This phenomenon of patient referral from the index hospital after BDI served further to confound obtaining adequate statistics on the true incidence of ductal injury.

Unfortunately, the use of IOC has continued to wane over the last 30 years. Early advocates for IOC have diminished especially in academic training programs where future surgeons should be trained in this procedure. This is especially notable since laparoscopic cholecystectomy is the most common procedure performed by surgical residents in the last several years [1]. For graduating surgical residents in 2018, laparoscopic cholecystectomy accounted for 11.2% of their operative cases (100 laparoscopic cholecystectomies throughout residency). Regarding the use of IOC in training programs, there has not been appropriate coding in resident case logs developed by the Accreditation Council on Graduate Medical Education (ACGME) to discern the true numbers of IOCs performed during residency training [1]. Unless IOC is supported and taught in surgical residency programs, this will be a lost skill, especially in the interpretation of an IOC by the surgeon.

Regarding common duct stones, an incidence of 10% of stones located outside the gallbladder has been well documented over many decades. If more than 700,000 cholecystectomies are performed each year in the United States annually, this translates to over 70,000 patients having CBD stones per annum. Before the laparoscopic era, well-trained surgeons successfully completed CBD stone removal in the first operative session and excellent results were published supporting this operative strategy. Despite surgical disciples who advocated for synchronous CBD stone management at the time of laparoscopic cholecystectomy, this surgical dictum has been virtually ignored in most clinical practices and training programs. The diminished use of the IOC has led to the increased incidence of retained ductal stones found after the index cholecystectomy. The avoidance of performing IOC and consequent reduction in surgical skill in managing ductal stones has been the result. Consequently, the reliance on endoscopic retrograde cholangiography (ERC) and sphincterotomy performed by gastroenterologists has been the result. This procedure has resulted in its own list of complications including perforation and bleeding (0.1–0.2%), and pancreatitis (5%). An additional consequence has been a loss of skill by younger surgeons in exploration of the common duct, extraction of stones and placement of T-tubes. Even in the scenario where an IOC is performed and the surgeon correctly interprets that CBD stones remain, these patients are often sent to nonsurgical colleagues for stone extraction in the postoperative period.

The lack of performance of IOC and avoidance of surgical management of identified CBD stones found at the time of laparoscopic cholecystectomy has not been lost on recent thought leaders. While it is vital that those surgeons currently performing biliary surgery embrace the principles of IOC and stone management, it is even more crucial that these principles be taught in the academic training programs where the future generations of surgeons are produced. These training programs must identify surgical champions who will be responsible for creation of a "Biliary Surgical Tract" in existing training programs in order to have trainees understand the importance of complete biliary stone management and to have the skill set necessary for the safe and complete surgical treatment of biliary stone disease.

It is also time to consider some significant improvements in patient care in order to decrease BDI and to enhance surgical removal of CBD stones during one operative setting.

The following recommendations would not interfere with existing training:

1. Introduction of strategies into the existing 5-year surgical residency training to enhance intraoperative visualization of the biliary system and CBD stone removal
2. Identify a subset of resident training programs that would incorporate these strategies into the 5-year curriculum
3. Encourage academic training programs to recruit faculty committed to teaching these strategies
4. Encourage use of the choledochoscope for removal of CBD stones under visual control at the time of LC
5. Mandate adequate record keeping and coding to document experience by trainees in the use of IOC and CBD stone extraction

What have we learned from our delving into history and the assessment of recent approaches to surgical management of biliary stone disease? These principles have taught us that we are constantly experiencing other examples of technological progress not only in surgical disciplines, but in all of health care. These newer and potentially disruptive technologies will need a measured and realistic evaluation before launching on the public. If we have learned anything, it is not to replicate a number of missteps experienced over the last 30 years in the introduction of laparoscopic surgical procedures. We will need a well thought-out structure that embraces the academic training programs for the evaluation of efficacy and safety and for the training of young surgeons in new techniques. The recent introduction of robotics into the surgical armamentarium requires this approach.

One does not have to be an economic expert to predict future changes in the healthcare system. Creation of new healthcare models is difficult and the path is strewn with failed examples [2]. There are already existing signs of future changes inherited from the past three decades which have only been heightened by the coronavirus pandemic of 2020. It is obvious that our capital investments for new costly procedures, complex instruments or technological outlays will be significantly scrutinized due to a decrease in the general health budget. We have to be realistic as we face a lower available health budget in the coming years; despite economic challenges, we must be vigilant in assuring safe outcomes for surgical patients.

One common misconception is that surgeons actually receive the amount of money billed for a surgical procedure! Patients have not realized that the reimbursement for a laparoscopic cholecystectomy may actually be one-third or less of the amount actually appearing in the billing statement. It is also a fact that a surgeon who is willing to perform an IOC during a cholecystectomy will probably not receive any significant additional reimbursement for adding this supplementary safety-related procedure.

Unlike hospital and operating room billing, additional time spent in the operating room by the operating surgeon is generally not a factor in surgical reimbursement. This additional time spent might actually be viewed as a negative when assigning surgeons to block time or positive incentives in ambulatory surgical centers or hospital operating suites. The incentive for attacking stones in the CBD is virtually nonexistent except for the satisfaction that a small fraction of surgeons derives from performing complete clearance of stones at one sitting. Even during times when a pandemic is affecting all healthcare sectors, movement has occurred to further reduce reimbursement for surgeons who participate in the federal programs of Medicare and Medicaid. Surgeons, like other humans, may need external incentives to achieve benchmarks. It would be ideal if internal incentives alone were a driving force.

Conclusion

Three decades ago, a completely new strategy was introduced for managing biliary stone disease. Decades later, it is obvious that the complications of BDI and retained CBD stones remain a significant problem. Why has this occurred? It occurred because important safeguards (IOC) were by-passed and that LC was separated from the CBD stone removal process. With improved strategies and incorporation of existing technology, mortality and morbidity can be decreased and difficult and painful postoperative complications (e.g., multiple operations) avoided.

Considering the last three decades of experience with laparoscopic surgery, it is illogical to believe that the current strategies followed by seasoned surgeons can be altered. Despite structured continuing medical education offerings by a multitude of professional organizations and academic centers, there has been movement away from the principles championed by Hans Kehr and others regarding management of biliary surgery and especially associated stones. Although there has been the development of hepatic and pancreatic (HPB) fellowships over the last several decades, the inclusion of training in laparoscopic gallbladder management has generally been left to the purview of surgeons not trained in HPB fellowships. More recently, "acute care" surgeons dedicated primarily to trauma management have been serving as attendings in academic training programs. If surgeons of the future are to have the will and skill to manage all aspects of gallbladder and stone disease, there must be mentors in academic centers who inculcate sound principles into their trainees. Since a surgical resident's most common operative experience is currently represented by laparoscopic cholecystectomy the same principles of HPB fellowship training could be woven into the general surgical training years. Through the efforts of groups such as the Safe Cholecystectomy Task Force, formed by SAGES in 2014, and the multidisciplinary group spawned from it, creating a consensus conference in 2018 and defined published recommendations in 2020 [3], solid proposals to enhance laparoscopic cholecystectomy have evolved. The ultimate goal now is to create programs to develop well-trained and complete biliary surgeons of the future. Deciding how best to move these proposals forward is a goal for us all.

References

1. Cortez AR, Potts JR. More of less: general surgery resident experience in biliary surgery. J Am Coll Surg, 2020, 231:33–42.
2. Toussaint JS. Why Haven healthcare failed. Harvard Business Review, 2021, Reprint H0647L.
3. Brunt LM, Deziel DJ, Telem DA, et al. Safe cholecystectomy multi-society practice guideline and state of the art consensus conference on prevention of bile duct injury during cholecystectomy. Ann Surg. 2020; 272: 3–23.

Correction to: No Stones Left Unturned

Correction to: G. Berci, F. L. Greene, *No Stones Left Unturned*,
https://doi.org/10.1007/978-3-030-76845-4

The below listed changes have been made in the corrected version of the book.
1. The frontispiece on the title page has been placed below the book title.
2. Affiliation for Dr. Bruce Gewertz has been updated in the front matter.
3. Chapter author's names had been missed out in chapters 14 and 17.
   Dr. J. Andrew Hamlin has been included as the author for chapter 14 and Professor Alfred Cuschieri has been included as the author for chapter 17.
4. On page 62, Chapter 8: The photographs of the early surgeons have been positioned in portrait position.
5. On page 80, Chapter 13: The photographs of the laparoscopic surgeons have been positioned in portrait position.

The updated online versions of the chapters can be found at
https://doi.org/10.1007/978-3-030-76845-4
https://doi.org/10.1007/978-3-030-76845-4_8
https://doi.org/10.1007/978-3-030-76845-4_13
https://doi.org/10.1007/978-3-030-76845-4_14
https://doi.org/10.1007/978-3-030-76845-4_17

© The Author(s), under exclusive license to Springer Nature Switzerland AG 2021
G. Berci, F. Greene, *No Stones Left Unturned*, https://doi.org/10.1007/978-3-030-76845-4_20

Index

A
Abdominal surgery, 57
Abdominal wall boil, 157
Academic surgeons, 128
Acute care surgery (ACS) services, 117, 118
American college of surgeons (ACS), 124
Anesthesia, 57
Antibiotic prophylaxis (AP), 97
Artificial intelligence (AI), 148

B
Berci, G., 77
Bile acids, 123
Bile duct exploration, 159
Bile duct injuries (BDI), 100, 153, 156, 166
    ductal-entero-anastomosis, 89
    operative cholangiograms, 88
    OR time extension, 87
    proximal hepatic system, 89
    slow injections, 88, 89
    small extravasations, 90
    surgeons, assistants, and nurses, 88
Biliary colic, 4
Biliary lithiasis, 131
Biliary stones
    carcinoma, 40, 42
    characteristic appearance, 35, 36
    choledochotomy and t-tube drainage, 36
    colicky pain, 37, 38
    empyema, 37
    hemorrhagic gallbladder, 37
    hydrops, 38
    mid-abdominal pain, 36
    preoperative position, 42
    right costal region, 38
    right upper quadrant pain, 38
Biliary surgery, 8, 155
    acute illness, 61
    choledocholithiasis, 121
    common duct, 61
    demonstrations, 8
    discovery, innovation and technological capability, 119
    ductus choledochus, 61
    evidence-based practices, 121
    general surgery residents graduation, 120, 121
    Glenn's biliary surgical cases, 62
    history, 119
    IOC, 121
    magnum opus, 8
    method of exploration, 9
    operation performance, 9
    operative procedures, 8
    patient's history, 9
    post-mortem specimens, 9
    residency training, 119
    right upper quadrant pain, 62
    SAGES, 119, 120
    training system, 8
    T-Tubes, 18, 19
    wound closure, 9
Bobbs, John Stough, 5

C
Carcinoma, 40, 42
Cholecystectomy, 137, 138
    abdominal surgery, 57
    clinical signs, 57
    common duct surgery, 57
    iodine deficiency, 57
    technique for, 57
Cholecystitis, 21
Cholecystolithiasis, 131
Cholecystostomy, 5
Choledocholithotomy, 91
Choledochoscope, 116
Cholelithiasis, 141
Chronica cholecystitis, 20
Common bile duct (CBD) stones, 91, 92
Convergence of disciplines, 127
Cosmesis, 116
Courvoisier, L., 57
Critical view of safety method, 146
Cystic duct, 24
    anatomical variations, 30
    configuration, 28
    hepatic artery, 31, 32
    malleable soft probe, 29

D
Diagnostic laparoscopy, 149
    cost, 150
    high income countrie, 149, 150
    history, 135
    incidence, 135
    intracorporeal techniques, 135
    investigation and bed turnover, 149
    manufacturer benefit, 150
    SAGES, 135, 136
    training equipment, 150
Disruptive technologies, 96, 127, 128
Dubois, F., 76

E
Electrocautery, 158
Endoscopic retrograde cholangiopancreatography (ERCP), 117, 131
Endoscopy
  common duct stone, 64
  diagnostic procedures, 64
  history, 53, 54
  innovation, 131, 132
  local manual manipulations, 65
  procedure, 64, 65
  teaching system, 65
Extracorporeal shockwave lithotripsy (ESWL), 115, 131
Extrahepatic bile ducts, 165

F
Flexible endoscopy, 147

G
Gallbladder surgery, 4, 5
Gallstone disease, 155
Gastric surgery, 61
General anesthesia, 137
Glenn, F., 62

H
Halsted, W.S., 61
Hepaticojejunostomy, 153
Hepatobiliary (HPB) fellowship, 153
Hopkins, H., 69
Hunter's principles, 126

I
Intraoperative cholangiography (IOCs), 127, 166–168
  benefits, 82
  biliary duct stones, 83
  biliary ductal anatomy, 82, 83
  injection cannula, 80
  operating room (OR), 81
  operative fluoro-cholangiography, 81, 82
Intraoperative fluorocholangiography (IOC), 121

J
Jacobeus, H.C., 54
Jaundice, 4

K
Kalk, H., 68
Kehr, Hans, 8–10
Kehr incisions, 44
  dilated choledochus, 46
  patient history, 47
  peritoneum, 45, 46
Kehr's attributes, 8
Ko, S.T., 77
Kocher, E.T., 57

L
Langenbuch, C.J.A., 57
Laparoscopic cholecystectomy (LC), 155, 157
  academic community, 124
  advantages, 138
  antibiotic prophylaxis, 97
  bile duct injury, 145, 146
  bile leaks, 98, 99
  clinical outcome, 97
  clinical research center, 142, 143
  complications recognition, 99
  conversion to open surgery, 97, 98
  day case/ambulatory LC
    benefits, 105
    bleeding complications, 105, 106
    patient outcome, 108
    robotically assisted surgery, 108
    on surgical practice, 106–108
    training and simulation, 106, 107
  ductal calculi, 103–105
  in elderly, 97
  falope loop, 123
  hernia repair, 124
  implementation, 124
  informed consent, 123
  instrumentation, 148
  MBDI, 100, 101
  miniature video camera, 123
  MVI, 101
  non-surgical treatment options, 138
  operative skills, 139
  origin, 96
  patient impact, 148
  performance, 141
  postoperative hospital stay, 97
  procedure, 76
  randomized clinical trials, 125, 126
  results, 77
  retrospective series, 99
  standard of care, 126
  surgical academic, 100
  surgical community, 138
  symptomatic gallstones, 103–105
  teaching attachment, 77
  techniques, 102, 103, 125, 126
  trainee reflections, 153, 154
  vascular injuries, 101, 102
Laparoscopic common bile duct exploration (LCBDE/LCDE), 117, 118, 128, 129
Laparoscopy, 68
  cysto- resectoscope, 70
  fiber bundle light conduction, 69
  monocular telescope, 71
  operative video endoscopy, 71
  TV camera, 71
  xenon light source, 70
Lumpectomy, 157

M
Major bile duct injuries (MBDI), 100, 101
Major vascular injuries (MVI), 101
Mastectomy, 157
Mayo, W., 61
Mini-cholecystectomy, 141
Minimal access surgery, 149
Minimally invasive surgery, 124
Mühe, E., 76

N
Nasobiliary (NB) drain, 98, 99
Nitze, M., 53

Index

O
Ohage, J.C., 62
Open cholecystectomy (OC), 98, 116, 128
Open Hasson technique, 101

P
Palliative care, 133
Pancreatitis, 158
Perforation, 158
Perrisat, J., 76
Petit, Jean-Louis, 4, 5
Phillips, E.H., 77
Piezoelectric extracorporeal shock wave lithotripsy, 119
Positive pressure capnoperitoneum, 101, 102
Postoperative pulmonary embolism, 76

R
Radiological access procedure, 115
Rectal disorders, 61
Reddick, E.J., 76
Robotic surgery, 129, 159
Ruddock, J.C., 68

S
Sims, J. Marion, 5
Society of American Gastrointestinal Endoscopic Surgeons (SAGES), 119, 120, 131, 135, 136
Storz, K., 70
Storz, S., 70
Stricture, 158

T
Tactile sensation, 157
Teaching programs, 165, 166
Technology development, 147
Thoracoscopy, 133
3-D technology, 115, 116
Training the trainers, 100

V
Vascular injury, 101, 102
Veress needle, 101, 138
Video-choledochoscopy, 65

W
Wildegans, H., 64

GPSR Compliance

The European Union's (EU) General Product Safety Regulation (GPSR) is a set of rules that requires consumer products to be safe and our obligations to ensure this.

If you have any concerns about our products, you can contact us on ProductSafety@springernature.com

In case Publisher is established outside the EU, the EU authorized representative is:

Springer Nature Customer Service Center GmbH
Europaplatz 3
69115 Heidelberg, Germany

Batch number: 08823285

Printed by Printforce, the Netherlands